# The Male Genitalia

## A CLINICIAN'S GUIDE TO SKIN PROBLEMS AND SEXUALLY TRANSMITTED INFECTIONS

**MANU SHAH**

*Consultant Dermatologist,*
*Dewsbury & District Hospital*
*West Yorkshire*
*United Kingdom*

with

**ARIYARATNE DE SILVA**

*Consultant in Genito-Urinary Medicine*
*Dewsbury & District Hospital*
*West Yorkshire*
*United Kingdom*

Radcliffe Publishing
Oxford • New York

**Radcliffe Publishing Ltd**
18 Marcham Road
Abingdon
Oxon OX14 1AA
United Kingdom

**www.radcliffe-oxford.com**

Electronic catalogue and worldwide online ordering facility.

British Library Cataloguing in Publication Data.

A catalogue record for this book is available from the British Library.

ISBN-13: 978 1 84619 040 7

Typeset by Pindar New Zealand (Egan Reid), Auckland, New Zealand
Printed and bound by Konway PrintHouse, Penang, Malaysia

# Contents

# Preface

Disease of the male genitalia is common, yet receives little in the way of publicity. Patients may be seen in primary care, genito-urinary medicine, dermatology or urology clinics. There is often little, if any, teaching of male genital disease in primary care.

Skin manifestations are very common in venereal infections. Emergence of HIV infection and the recent resurgence of syphilis demonstrate the importance of having a quick reference guide available for physicians in both primary and secondary care.

Over the last decade we have developed excellent networking between the dermatology and the genito-urinary medicine departments in Dewsbury. Working together closely has improved patient care immensely and has enabled us to compile this presentation.

The book covers the broad area of male genital disease encompassing dermatology and genito-urinary medicine. It will serve as a quick reference guide for dermatologists, genito-urinary medicine physicians and will be useful to medical students, doctors in primary care and those running specialty clinics for sexual health.

At a time when the rate of sexually transmitted diseases is rising rapidly in both developed and under-developed nations and public awareness of sexual health is increasing, we feel the timing of a book on male genital problems is appropriate.

**Manu Shah**
*September 2007*

# About the authors

**Manu Shah** is consultant dermatologist at Dewsbury & District Hospital in West Yorkshire. He has a special interest in skin cancer and runs a specialist clinic for men with genital skin problems.

**Ariyaratne De Silva** is consultant in genito-urinary medicine at Dewsbury & District Hospital. He leads an award-winning department which is the first and only genito-urinary service nationally to be recognised for the Charter Mark (excellence in customer care) three times.

# Acknowledgements

We wish to thank our many patients who have kindly agreed to allow the publication of their photographs. Dr A Jackson helped photograph a number of microscopic sections. The staff in the dermatology and genito-urinary medicine departments in Dewsbury have been very supportive. Dr N Cox, Dr KN Sankar and Dr GJ Sobey have kindly given helpful comments. The staff of Dewsbury and District Hospital Staff Library have been a source of constant help and support.

All the graphs have been redrawn but with the public health data provided by the Health Protection Agency in the United Kingdom.

# Disclaimer

New research and clinical experience can result in changes in treatment and drug therapy. Readers of this book should therefore check the most recent product information on any drug they may prescribe to ensure they are complying with the manufacturer's recommendations concerning dosage, the method and duration of administration, and contraindications. Neither the publisher nor the author accept liability for any injury or damage arising from this publication.

# 1

# Anatomy and normal variants, history taking and basic examination

Before attempting to diagnose male genital skin problems it is important to know the normal anatomy of the genitalia and how to take a detailed history specific to genital problems.

In this chapter we will look at:
- normal anatomy of the male genitalia
- normal anatomical variants commonly seen
- taking a dermatological and sexual history
- examination of the male genitalia
- tests performed in the dermatology clinic
- basic screening tests performed in the setting of the genito-urinary medicine clinic.

## NORMAL ANATOMY

The anatomy of the male genitalia varies greatly between individuals and it is important for doctors to recognise this, especially when reassuring anxious patients. The development of a genital skin problem may result in the first detailed self-inspection of a man's genitalia.

Knowledge of the topographical anatomy of the male genitalia is useful, particularly when describing location of lesions. The ventral aspect of the penis is the underside surface continuous with the scrotum (*see* Figure 1.1).

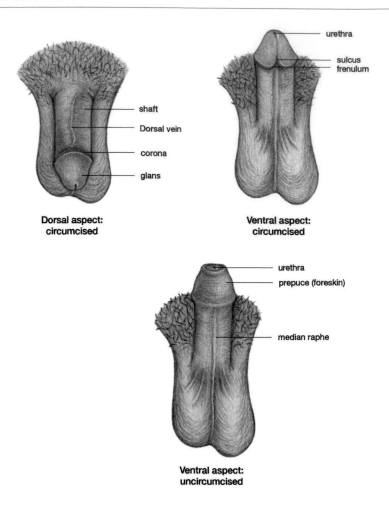

**FIGURE 1.1** Normal anatomy of the male genitalia.

## NORMAL ANATOMICAL VARIANTS

**TABLE 1.1** The commonest anatomical variants and lesions of the male genitalia

|  | See also |
| --- | --- |
| Angiokeratomas | Chapter 5, page 55 |
| Hyper/hypopigmentation | Chapter 7, page 77 |
| Naevi | Chapter 5, page 47 |
| Pearly penile papules | *See* below |
| Prominent veins | *See* below |
| Sebaceous prominence | *See* below |
| Skin tags | Chapter 5, page 53 |

## Pearly penile papules (*see* Figure 4.2, page 39)

This common variant consists of asymptomatic papules (histologically these are angiofibromas) running around the coronal sulcus. They occur in all racial groups and are seen in approximately one in five men. They may be confused with viral warts if filiform in nature.

## Prominent veins

Prominent veins may be visible on the scrotum, the shaft of the penis or the prepuce. Their presence may occasionally cause anxiety.

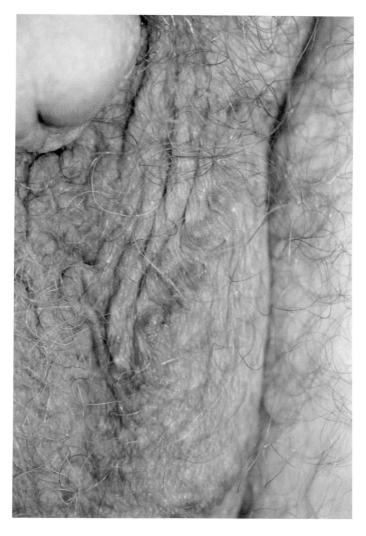

FIGURE 1.2 Prominent veins on the scrotum. A common finding.

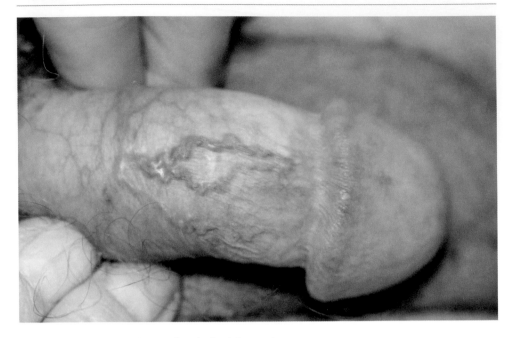

**FIGURE 1.3** Prominent veins on the shaft of the penis.

## Hyper/hypopigmentation

Genital pigmentation is very common and is discussed in more detail in Chapter 7.

## Sebaceous prominence/hyperplasia

This common finding represents enlarged or prominent sebaceous glands in the skin. They are often visible around the shaft of the penis and the foreskin and are usually just a millimetre or less in size.

## TAKING A DERMATOLOGICAL AND SEXUAL HISTORY

It is important to ask questions that are both relevant and sensitive. In the dermatological part of the history the following information is needed:

- presenting symptoms – rash, itch, lesion, soreness, etc.
- duration of problems
- concurrent illness especially skin disorders, e.g. psoriasis, eczema
- previous skin conditions, e.g. eczema, psoriasis, lichen planus
- medication – current and previous including topical agents
- whether the patient is a smoker
- occupation.

**FIGURE 1.4** Median raphe of the scrotum. This one is hypopigmented. The median raphe represents the midline fusion of ectoderm during embryogenesis.

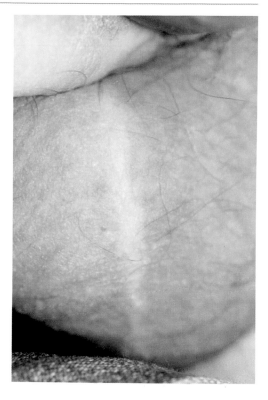

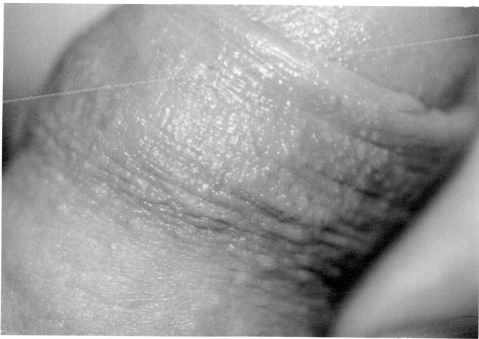

**FIGURE 1.5** Sebaceous prominence of the foreskin.

When taking a sexual history it is important to remember that sexually transmitted infections are increasing rapidly in most countries in the world and common, important infections like chlamydia may remain asymptomatic. Sexually transmitted infections are more frequently found among young people and the offer of screening tests for common infections is beneficial in most health care settings. In taking a sexual history the following points may prove useful:

- reassurance with regards to confidentiality is essential
- the need for taking a sexual history should be explained
- the health care professional should not be embarrassed to ask vital questions that would help in taking the appropriate tests and making an accurate diagnosis
- it is a good habit to warn the patient that you are going to ask some sensitive questions
- attitude should be non-judgmental
- do not make assumptions on sexuality, behaviour and practices
- use terms that the individual would understand and interpret properly
- ideally, the sexual history should be taken on a one-to-one level, but respect the patient's view if a third person is requested to reduce anxiety.

The following questions would make up a detailed sexual history in the male:

- type of symptoms and duration (with relation to the last sexual contact)
- any urethral discharge?
- symptoms of dysuria?
- pain, lumps or swellings in the genital area/groins/scrotum
- any ulceration/blisters? If so, are they painful or painless?
- recent genital or generalised rashes?
- itching/soreness of the genitals?
- date of most recent sexual contact (beware of the 'window' period)
- details of the partner, i.e.  Male/Female
  Regular/casual/prostitute
  Where local/abroad
- anatomical areas that were exposed to sexual contact; urethral, pharynx, rectum
- was a condom used – throughout/all exposures?
- other sexual contacts in the last three months?
- number of sexual contacts in the last twelve months (risk assessment)
- past sexually transmitted infections
- risk factors: use of drugs (intravenous)/alcohol.

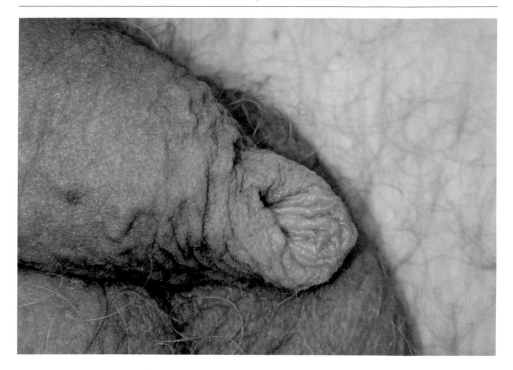

**FIGURE 1.6** Long, flaccid foreskin (normal variant).

## EXAMINATION OF THE MALE GENITALIA

The genitals should be examined in a systematic fashion. Tattoos and piercings are relatively common and may be associated with disease, such as an increased risk of infective hepatitis and other infections. The penis, scrotum, mons pubis and groins should be examined in turn. The following system may be helpful during examination.

### Penis

- Examine the shaft, noting skin lesions and any structural abnormalities, tenderness or plaques.
- Inspect the glans penis (first fully retract foreskin) noting the position of the meatus and the median raphe (deviated to the left side in 10% of men).
- Coronal area of the glans: a common area for inflammatory skin disease.
- Meatus – look for stricture, inflammation, viral warts.
- Look for a urethral discharge; notice the colour and the consistency if present.
- Inspect the frenulum (small warts may be missed if present in this region).

### Scrotum
- Palpate the testis (should have a firm consistency, around 4 × 6cm in size).
- Palpate epididymis.
- Examine the skin of the scrotum.

### Mons pubis
- Look for hair abnormalities and signs of infestation.

### Groins
- Move the skin folds to reveal the skin of the groins and observe for signs of disease (*see* Chapter 2).
- Palpate the inguinal nodes to see if they are enlarged. Note the size, presence of tenderness and consistency of any nodes.


## TESTS PERFORMED IN THE DERMATOLOGY CLINIC

The majority of patients presenting to the dermatology clinic with a genital problem do not have a sexually transmitted infection. Tests are therefore directed at screening for skin conditions. The Wood's (ultraviolet) light is used to look for areas of skin that may fluoresce. This may occur with certain bacterial and fungal infections. Microbiological swabs are often taken from the groins and glans penis, particularly looking for evidence of candida and anaerobic bacterial infection. Where fungal disease is suspected skin scrapings from scaly lesions may be taken, then sent for mycological analysis. The most important test available to dermatologists is the skin biopsy with histological analysis.

Skin biopsies taken from the male genitalia may be necessary to exclude malignant and pre-malignant conditions and to diagnose inflammatory skin disease. The genital skin is highly vascular and heals quickly following biopsy.


## SCREENING MEN IN THE GENITO-URINARY CLINIC SETTING

Screening tests for men with potential sexually transmitted diseases vary from country to country. The tests performed must be in proportion to the risk a patient has subjected himself to and how useful investigation will be in the management. The number of tests may be limited by local resources. Tests may be available locally for detecting these conditions:
- chlamydia trachomatis and lymphogranuloma venereum
- syphilis
- gonorrhoea
- candidosis and other yeast and fungal infections

- HIV 1 & 2
- viral hepatitis
- herpes simplex infection.

A standard low-cost set of screening investigations may include the following:
- a small cotton wool or plastic loop can take a urethral specimen which is smeared onto a microscope slide for gram-staining
- the same loop is used to plate directly onto a selective medium for N gonorrhoeae
- a two-glass urine test can be performed to exclude urethritis: the patient passes urine into two clean specimen glasses (10–20ml in the first and the rest into the second). If the urine is hazy, 5% acetic acid is added until all phosphate crystals are dissolved. In the presence of pus in the anterior urethra, the haze will persist in the first glass due to pus cells, threads or flecks and the second glass will remain clear
- the first urine specimen can be tested for chlamydia by using a nucleic acid amplification test. If this is not available a fine urethral swab can be inserted 1–2cm into the urethra to take a sample for chlamydia trachomatis

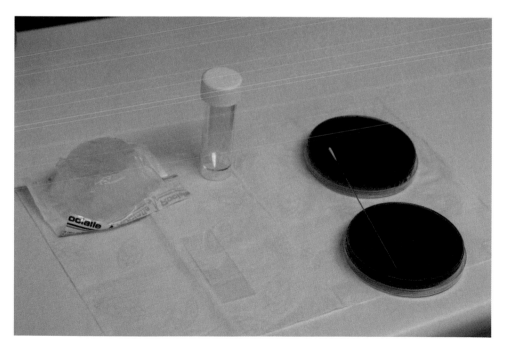

**FIGURE 1.7** Basic equipment for screening male patients (collection dish for urine, sample bottle, agar plates, microscope slide and penile swab).

- blood test for syphilis serology
- a mid-stream urine sample may be necessary to exclude a urinary tract infection
- other specific tests may be performed depending on the clinical situation and risk (e.g. blood test for hepatitis, HIV etc).

## KEY POINTS

❭ Normal variations in the anatomy of the male genitalia are common but may cause confusion and anxiety in patients and doctors.

❭ A careful and sensitive dermatological and sexual history is important in patients with genital symptoms.

❭ A systematic examination of the genitalia is essential.

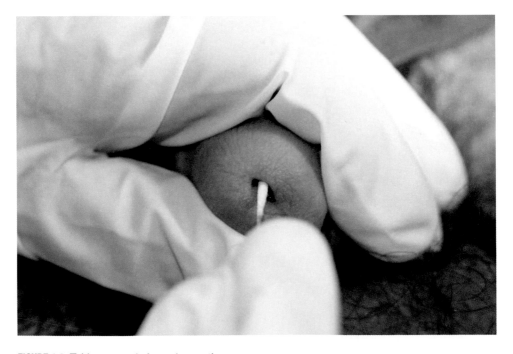

**FIGURE 1.8** Taking a swab from the urethra.

**CASE STUDY**

John, a 17-year-old at college, had been worried about some 'warts' on the glans penis after having had sex for the first time. He was too embarrassed to ask his general practitioner about them so made an appointment at the local genito-urinary medicine clinic. He was much relieved to discover that what he feared as warts were actually called pearly penile papules and are a common, normal finding in many men.

# 2

# Hair and groin problems

A number of inflammatory dermatoses and infective conditions commonly affect the groin areas, as well as the hair-bearing areas and peri-anal region. These problems may present to the sexual health clinic or may be seen in the general practice setting or the dermatology department. They may be a primary problem or a complication of a more general disorder. Diseases affecting the hairy areas and groins most commonly seen are:

1. Intertrigo.
2. Tinea cruris.
3. Erythrasma.
4. Folliculitis.
5. Alopecia areata.
6. Hydradenitis suppurativa.
7. Pubic lice (*see* Chapter 3, page 31).

## 1. INTERTRIGO

Intertrigo is an inflammatory dermatosis of skin folds. It may be caused or complicated by yeast, bacterial or fungal infection.

## Incidence

Intertrigo is a common condition, affecting all races, and is particularly found in old people and young children. It is more common in hot and humid environments.

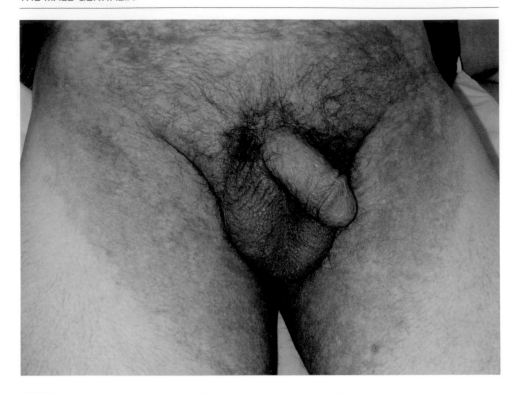

**FIGURE 2.1** An acute contact dermatitis causing extensive intertrigo.

### Clinical history and examination

The usual presenting symptoms are of chronic irritation of the skin folds with itching and burning being prominent symptoms.

The skin tends to be erythematous, macerated and can be crusted. Any skin folds can be affected but commonly problems occur in abdominal folds, groin creases and peri-anal areas.

### Candidosis as a cause of intertrigo

Candidosis (infection due to the yeast candida albicans) is the commonest cause of intertrigo. Clinical examination reveals red plaques in the skin folds, often with small erosions. Pustules may also be visible and there may be evidence of balanoposthitis (inflammation of the glans penis and prepuce).

There are a number of predisposing causes of candidosis, including diabetes mellitus, urinary incontinence, obesity, the use of systemic antibiotics, iron deficiency and conditions where the immune system is suppressed, such as HIV infection.

**TABLE 2.1** Causes of genito-crural intertrigo

| Common causes | | See also | Rare causes | |
|---|---|---|---|---|
| **Infective** | Candidosis | Below | Inflammatory | Reiter's syndrome (*see* Chapter 6) |
| | Tinea | Below | | Darier's disease |
| | Erythrasma | Below | | Lichen sclerosus (Chapter 4) |
| | | | | Hailey-Hailey disease (below) |
| **Inflammatory** | Psoriasis | Chapter 11, page 120 | Malignant | Extra-mammary Paget's disease (below) |
| | Irritant & contact dermatitis | Chapter 11, page 124 | | Bowens disease (Chapter 5) |
| | Seborrhoeic eczema | Chapter 11, page 127 | | |

## Diagnosis of intertrigo

The diagnosis of intertrigo can be made clinically but a cause must be sought. Wood's (ultraviolet) light examination of the groin area will exclude erythrasma

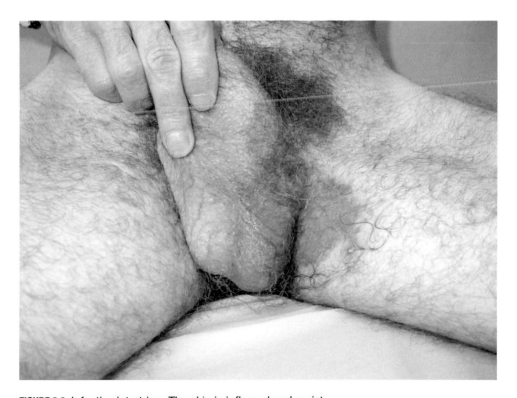

**FIGURE 2.2** Infective intertrigo. The skin is inflamed and moist.

(page 20). Skin scrapings should be taken for microscopy and mycological culture to exclude tinea and yeast infection. Microbiological swabs should be performed to exclude bacterial infection. For persistent problems a skin biopsy may be necessary, particularly to exclude rare causes of genito-crural intertrigo (Table 2.1). Patch testing looking for contact allergy may also be necessary (e.g. for the patient in Figure 2.1), and is important if the inflammatory problem also affects the peri-anal area. Underlying conditions that will pre-dispose the patient to intertrigo, such as diabetes, should be excluded.

## Treatment

### a. General advice

Treating underlying problems is essential in the management of intertrigo. Correction of metabolic disease, especially diabetes, is important. Good hygiene can often solve the problem, and may be an issue for incontinent patients. Daily washing is essential, but harsh antiseptic agents should be avoided. Emollient washes are soothing and non-irritant. Where obesity causing excessive skin folds can not be improved by dietary measures, the skin should be separated with dressings and kept dry. Barrier creams may be useful.

### b. Specific measures

For infective problems antimycotic agents (e.g. topical clotrimazole, itraconazole) and anti-infective agents (antiseptics, topical antibiotics for short-term use) may prove useful. For inflammatory dermatoses a topical steroid will be necessary in the short-term (there is a risk of skin atrophy in skin folds with longer-term use). Often a combined steroid-anti-infective agent cream is necessary due to the presence of secondary infection.

## 2. TINEA CRURIS

Tinea cruris is a superficial dermatophyte infection of the groin and pubic area.

## Incidence

Tinea cruris is extremely common, being three times more common in men than women. It reaches peak incidence in men aged 18–25 and 40–50 years. Epidemics may occur in schools and other institutions, where contaminated towels, pool areas and showers are to blame.

## Clinical history and examination

Tinea cruris invariably presents as an itchy rash in the groin. It is exacerbated by wearing tight fitting or wet clothing. Poor hygiene, obesity and diabetes mellitus may be implicated.

The rash presents as an erythematous eruption, often with a sharply demarcated periphery with scale. Typically, there is central clearing of the rash. The penis and scrotum may be affected in more extensive infection. Due to the chronic itch, secondary lichenified eczema is common, resulting from scratching. At least 50% of patients will have co-existing tinea pedis.

## Complicating factors

Tinea may be found in other sites such as the nails, the feet, the peri-anal area and on the body. It may be extremely difficult to diagnose if it has been modified by the use of topical corticosteroids (then called 'tinea incognito'). The rash then looks non-specific, often eczematous but without the scaly edge.

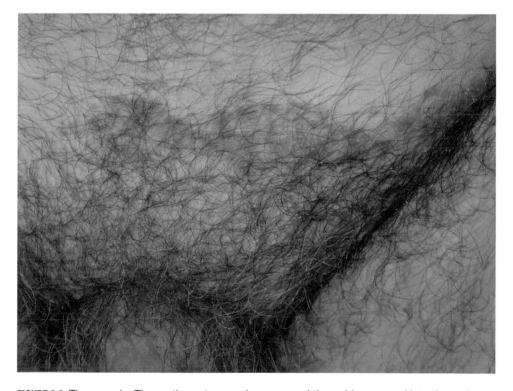

**FIGURE 2.3** Tinea cruris. The erythematous rash runs round the pubic area and into the groin.

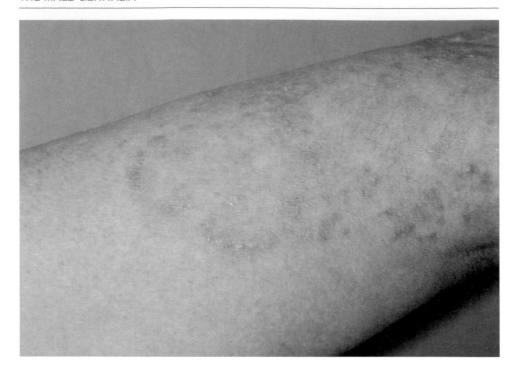

**FIGURE 2.4** Tinea. Note the scaly edge of the rash.

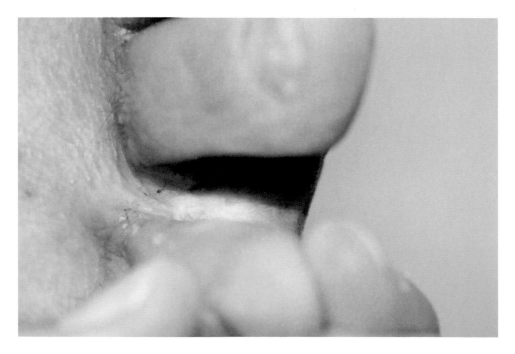

**FIGURE 2.5** Tinea pedis – white macerated skin between the toes.

## Diagnosis

Wood's light examination will exclude erythrasma (*see* page 20). Skin scrapings from the edge of a lesion when viewed under the microscope should show fungal hyphae and spores. The skin scrapings should also be sent for fungal culture. Where tinea has not been excluded and skin biopsy is performed, a PAS stain may show dermatophytes in the stratum corneum.

## Treatment

As with all causes of intertrigo, underlying problems such as obesity and diabetes should be corrected if possible. General measures such as avoiding tight fitting clothing and keeping the groin dry are necessary. Auto-inoculation from tinea on the feet is common, usually through towel use. Separate towels for the groin and the rest of the body should be used. For mild infections, topical antifungal agents such as ketoconazole and terbinafine can be used. For more extensive eruptions and in ano-genital dermatophytosis, oral treatments with terbinafine or itraconazole will be necessary. Where re-infection occurs (in about 20% of cases), it is important to look for dermatophyte infection of the feet that has been inadequately treated.

## Rare causes of intertrigo

### Extra-mammary Paget's disease

This rare malignant disease is a differential diagnosis in unusual forms of intertrigo. It is an indolent adenocarcinoma mainly affecting elderly people. It may present as a chronic irritating and itchy rash, usually a reddish-brown plaque, anywhere in the ano-genital region. It is often mis-diagnosed as an inflammatory dermatosis such as eczema or psoriasis, and it is not uncommon for there to be a delay in diagnosis of several years.

Skin biopsy is essential to diagnose the condition. The disease occurs as scaly, moist inflammatory plaques that are locally invasive and have metastatic potential. A proportion of patients will have a co-existing underlying malignant disease, such as an adenocarcinoma of the gastrointestinal or urogenital tract. Surgical excision is the treatment of choice. Extensive disease may respond to topical 5-fluouracil.

### Hailey-Hailey disease (benign familial pemphigus)

This is an autosomal dominant condition characterised by scaly or vegetative plaques of the flexures. It usually presents at around 10 to 30 years of age. Lesions may appear moist or scaly. Pustules and vesicles are usually present. The lesions appear very similar to the flexural lesions of Darier's disease and there is some clinical overlap between these two genetic disorders.

The diagnosis may be difficult and should be considered in any form of intertrigo unresponsive to therapy. Diagnosis should be confirmed by skin biopsy.

## 3. ERYTHRASMA

Erythrasma is a common, chronic infection of the skin folds, particularly the groin and axillary areas. It is caused by a bacterium called Corynebacterium minutissimum.

### Incidence

The incidence of erythrasma has been reported in various studies from between 0.5% and 4% of the population. It is more frequently found in subtropical and tropical areas of the world and is more common with high humidity.

### Clinical history and examination

Erythrasma is often recognised incidentally since it is usually asymptomatic. It may occasionally be pruritic. There are a number of predisposing factors which include hyperhydrosis, obesity, diabetes mellitus and other conditions where the immune system is compromised.

It presents as a pink or brown discolouration of the skin of flexures associated with some dryness of the skin. While it is usually confined to the flexures, it may occasionally involve extensive areas of the body.

### Diagnosis of erythrasma

The diagnosis of erythrasma is easily made using the Wood's light. Under this light the affected skin fluoresces a coral pink colour (due to porphyrins released by the bacteria). A gram stain performed on skin biopsy will often reveal gram positive rods of the diptheroid bacteria.

### Treatment

As with other forms of intertrigo, erythrasma should be initially treated by hygiene measures and managing underlying conditions such as obesity and diabetes. Topical treatment with antibiotics or antiseptic therapies is successful.

However, for more extensive infection or infection resistant to topical treatment, oral erythromycin or oral tetracycline can be used.

## 4. FOLLICULITIS

Folliculitis is an inflammation of hair follicles most often caused by infection. In men, the most common cause is infection with staphylococcus aureus. Folliculitis is also very common as a result of trauma and irritation, particularly due to shaving in the groin area. Folliculitis is more common in patients with immuno-suppression, particularly those suffering from diabetes.

### Incidence

Folliculitis is extremely common in both men and women. Certain types of folliculitis are more common in certain groups of men. For example, pseudomonas folliculitis may be acquired from contaminated hot tubs. Eosinophilic, pustular folliculitis is seen in patients with HIV disease (*see* Chapter 10).

### Clinical history and examination

Patients complain of an itchy pustular rash, usually of the thighs and groins.

The lesion most commonly found in folliculitis is an erythematous papule or pustule centred around a hair. The hair shaft in the middle of the lesion may have been lost and hence is not always visible.

### Diagnosis of folliculitis

The clinical diagnosis of folliculitis is usually easy as pustules are the commonest feature. Predisposing factors should be looked for, particularly problems with excess sweating, use of topical corticosteroids, staphylococcal nasal carrier patients and patients with immune deficiencies (including diabetes and HIV). Folliculitis may simply be caused by irritant factors such as friction, occlusion and shaving. Infective causes need to be excluded. Microbiological swabs will exclude bacterial infections. Pus from a lesion can be examined for evidence of fungal infection and a viral swab may be useful to exclude herpes simplex folliculitis (although this is rare).

### Treatment

As with the treatment for intertrigo, daily washing is essential, particularly with

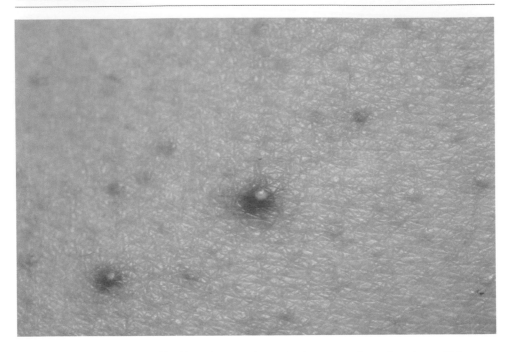

**FIGURE 2.6** Lesions of folliculitis. Note the pustule centred on an erythematous base. Hairs are not visible.

anti-bacterial cleansers. Systemic antibiotics may be necessary and these should have activity against staphylococcus aureus. For patients with staphylococcus aureus carriage the organism needs to be eliminated from the nose and the skin. There is evidence to support the use of topical antibiotics, although these should be used for limited periods to prevent the development of bacterial resistance.

For the treatment of unusual forms of folliculitis, different therapies may also be necessary. Pseudomonas folliculitis should respond to oral ciprofloxacin, pityrosporum folliculitis will respond to systemic antifungal agents (e.g. ketoconazole) and herpetic folliculitis should respond to an appropriate anti-viral agent such as aciclovir, famciclovir or valaciclovir.

## 5. ALOPECIA AREATA

It is worth mentioning this common form of hair loss since it may affect the genital area. It is rare for alopecia areata just to affect the pubic hair and signs of hair loss should be looked for elsewhere. Classically, the area of hair loss is well-circumscribed. It is worth remembering that there are many causes of hair loss, including syphilis.

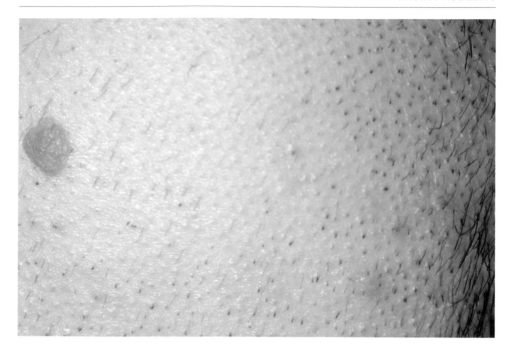

**FIGURE 2.7** Alopecia areata. Note the naevus on the left.

## 6. HYDRADENITIS SUPPURATIVA

Hydradenitis suppurativa is a chronic, relapsing spectrum of diseases characterised by folliculitis, comedones and deep, discharging sinuses, cysts, fistulae and scars.

### Incidence

The condition is less common in men compared with women. The incidence in the general population may be up to 4%. The condition usually presents after puberty and is particularly common in the second and third decades of life.

### Clinical history and examination

Patients may complain of recurrent infections and boils in the genital area. Lesions may be itchy and are often tender.

The most common affected area in men is the perineum (compared with the axillae in women). The condition may present with a variety of signs, including folliculitis, cysts, nodules and scars in the groins, axillae and perineum. Scarring may be extensive and may interfere with sexual activity. Examination may reveal

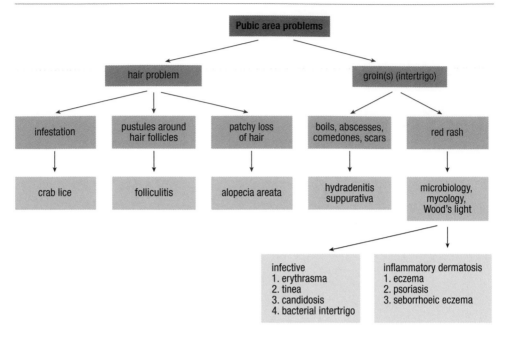

**FIGURE 2.8** Flow chart to aid diagnosis of common problems in the pubic area.

open comedones ('blackheads') and pili incarnati (in-growing hairs). Mild disease may present as isolated tender or pruritic nodules in the groins or perineum. With worsening disease, subcutaneous extension leads to a chronic suppurative condition. Discharging abscesses and sinuses may then occur. Local lymph node swelling is usually absent even with severe disease. Cystic acne and Crohn's disease are differential diagnoses and may need to be excluded.

## Diagnosis of hydradenitis suppurativa

Diagnosis is made clinically in the vast majority of patients. Where other conditions such as Crohn's disease are suspected, skin biopsy and other investigations may be helpful. Diabetes should be excluded since it may be a complicating factor. Routine microbiological tests may reveal a variety of bacteria, particularly staphylococcus aureus, streptococci and *E coli*.

## Treatment

For mild disease short courses of antibiotics for two to three weeks may suffice. A range of antibiotics have been shown to be beneficial. These include tetracyclines, flucloxacillin, metronidazole, ciprofloxacin and clindamycin. For more severe disease, especially of the chronic, relapsing type long-term antibiotics (many months) may be necessary. Systemic steroids may be useful in short courses to reduce the inflammatory process. Other options include systemic retinoid drugs (e.g. isotretinoin). Surgical resection of diseased and scarred tissue may be helpful in extensive disease where there are persistent localised problems.

## Complications

Many of the complications of hydradenitis suppurativa lead to a reduced quality of life for sufferers. Continually discharging abscesses and sinuses can lead to a chronic anaemia and psychological and psychosexual problems. There is a rare association with squamous cell carcinoma for disease lasting over 20 years. Fistulae formation has been described occurring into the urethra, bladder and rectum. Chronic localised lymphoedema may occur and give rise to swellings of the penis and scrotum.

## 7. PUBIC LICE (*see* Chapter 3, page 31)

## KEY POINTS

» Intertrigo is a clinical sign, not a diagnosis. Causes should be sought.
» The commonest cause of intertrigo is candida infection.
» General hygiene measures are important in the management of all hair and groin problems.
» Fungal, yeast and bacterial infection commonly complicate pubic hair and groin problems.

---

### CASE STUDY

Max was a keen sportsman who was severely troubled by 'jock itch'. This flared intermittently. He had tried many over the counter preparations without success. When examined he had severe tinea pedis and widespread tinea around the groin and perianal areas. He responded rapidly to oral terbinafine. He was given detailed advice on preventing re-infection.

# 3

# Genital itching

There are many causes of genital itching but they can be divided into the following three groups of conditions:

1. Genital itch as a part of a skin disorder.
   - Irritant dermatitis            *see* Chapter 11, page 124.
   - Seborrhoeic dermatitis     *see* Chapter 11, page 127.
   - Psoriasis                  *see* Chapter 11, page 120.
   - Contact dermatitis         *see* Chapter 11, page 123.
   - Lichen planus              *see* Chapter 6, page 69.
   - Lichen sclerosus           *see* Chapter 1, page 38.
   - Scabies                    *see* below.
2. Localised genital infection, infestations and bites.
   - Candida                    *see* Chapter 2, page 14.
   - Tinea                       *see* Chapter 2, page 16.
   - Erythrasma              *see* Chapter 2, page 20.
   - Scabies                    *see* below.
   - Pubic lice                *see* below.
   - Insect bites             *see* below.
3. Psychogenic causes (*see* Chapter 12).
   - Psychosexual problems     *see* page 129.
   - Delusions of parasitosis    *see* page 131.
   - Burning scrotum syndrome etc.   *see* page 129.

This chapter is concerned with arthropods (insects, spiders and mites) as a cause of genital itching. This is an important topic particularly in young men where the prevalence of sexually transmitted infections is highest. The other causes of genital itching are covered elsewhere in this book.

## SCABIES

Scabies is a common infestation of the skin caused by the mite sarcoptes scabiei. The majority of cases of scabies are not sexually transmitted. However, the genitals are the third most common body site affected by scabies. Genital itching due to scabies is a common reason why patients attend sexual health clinics.

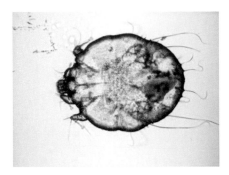

**FIGURE 3.1** Enlargement of a scabies mite. The actual size is approximately 0.3mm.

### Incidence

Scabies occurs in all populations. It affects millions of people on a world wide basis and often occurs in epidemics. No racial group is immune to infestation. Sexually-active people and the immuno-compromised have a higher risk of infection. There is evidence that sexually transmitted scabies is becoming more common but unfortunately most countries (including the UK and US) do not have centrally collected data. However, the number of people attending sexual health clinics who are diagnosed as having scabies is rising.

### Clinical history and examination

The main symptom is itch which is invariably more intense at night time. Patients will often give a history of contact with someone who is also itching.

The clinical signs may be variable. The major physical sign is a short serpiginous burrow. The burrow is a tunnel within the stratum corneum with the mite present at the blind end. Burrows tend to be around 4 to 5mm long. The location of the mite may be determined by the presence of a tiny black dot or small elevation surrounded by a red ring at one end of the burrow. Vesicles, papules or pustules may also develop where mites are present.

Red papules on the glans penis, shaft of the penis and the scrotum are said to be pathognomonic of scabies in men. It is unusual for scabies just to affect

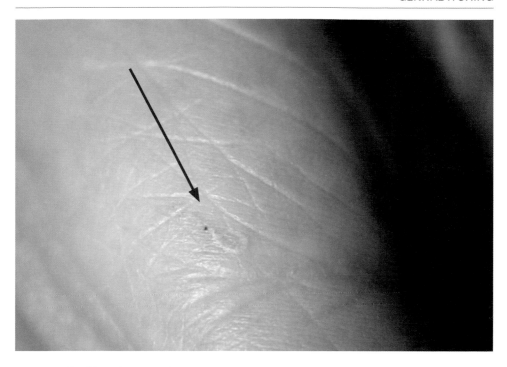

FIGURE 3.2 Scabies of the hand showing a short almost circular burrow with small black dot (the mite) at one end (arrow).

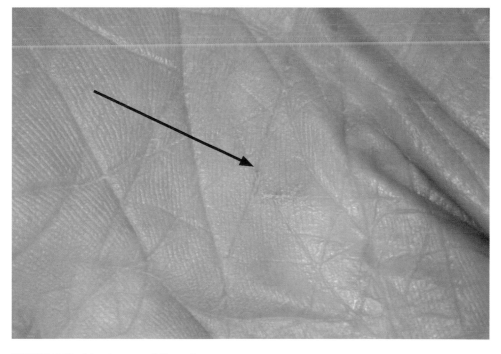

FIGURE 3.3 Scabies burrow of the palm.

the genitals and other body sites will almost certainly be affected. Burrows can often be detected in the web spaces of the fingers, the flexures, axillae, umbilicus, buttocks and the feet.

The diagnosis of scabies can be extremely difficult if burrows are not visible. There are only around 10–15 mites on average. Burrows are often scratched, changing their appearance. It is not uncommon for patients with scabies to develop secondary bacterial infection and eczema due to constant scratching. Again, these secondary signs may disguise or destroy burrows. In addition, patients may have been treated with anti-pruritic agents and topical steroids. This tends to alter the appearance of the rash.

Crusted or Norwegian scabies is a rare form of the disease in which individuals become infected with millions of mites, usually due to a reduced immunological response. This form of the disease is highly infectious.

## Treatment

All household members and close personal and sexual contacts should be treated whether or not they exhibit signs or itch. Topical therapies have to be left on

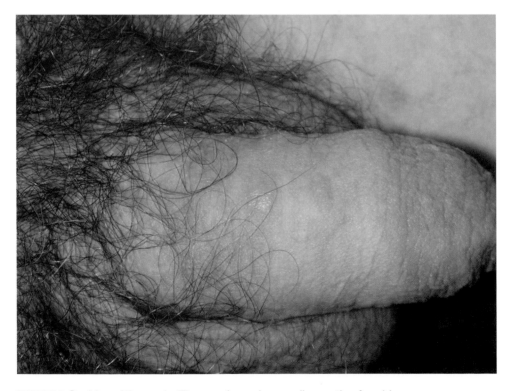

**FIGURE 3.4** Scabies of the penis. These red papules are diagnostic of scabies.

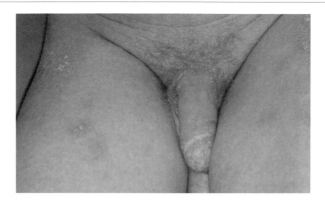

**FIGURE 3.5** Norwegian or crusted scabies of the glans penis.

for prolonged periods. Treatment failures may occur if therapies are washed off (e.g. from the hands) and not re-applied. The following topical therapies have all been used:

- permethrin 5% single application, left on for 8 to 12 hours
- lindane 1% single application, left on for 8 to 12 hours (not available in some European countries due to possible neurological side effects)
- malathion 0.5%. Comes as both an aqueous and an alcoholic product. Single application. Applied all over and washed off after 24 hours.
- benzyl benzoate 25% applied on three successive days for 24 hours each day (rarely used)
- sulphur 6–33% applied on three successive days for 24 hours each day (rarely used)
- scabies is acquired from close physical contact and the decision must be made to offer screening for sexually transmitted infections if this is appropriate.

## PUBIC LICE (SYN. PHTHIRUS PUBIS, PEDICULOSIS PUBIS)

The pubic or crab louse is a human parasite, measuring around 1–2mm in diameter. The adult louse varies from light brown to dark grey in colour. The name comes from the crab-like claws that are used to clasp hairs whilst the mouth parts are buried in the skin to suck blood. The life cycle is about 15–20 days. The incubation period of the egg is around five days. Transmission occurs through skin contact and up to 95% of sexual contacts of an index patient may acquire the infestation.

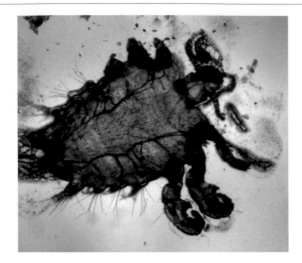

**FIGURE 3.6** Close up view of a pubic louse.

## Incidence

The condition tends to occur sporadically. It affects all racial groups. It is more common in cooler months in contrast to body and head lice, which tend to be commoner in the warmer months. The incidence rates for pubic lice in both the US and UK have been estimated at approximately 1 in 90 with around 3 200 000 cases in the US and 665 000 cases in the UK (US Census Bureau 2004).

## Clinical history and examination

Patients most often present with genital itching, usually worse at night. However, it is not usual for asymptomatic cases to be discovered during routine examination at sexual health clinics.

The following physical signs may be evident:

- erythema and scratch marks
- adult lice attached to hairs
- eggs (nits). Adult lice and eggs are most often found in the pubic region but in hairy men they may be as widespread as the thighs, trunk, axillae and eyelashes
- minute blood stains in the patient's underwear
- 'black powder' which represents insect faecal matter may also be visible in the patient's underwear.
- signs of secondary infection
- occasional inguinal lymphadenopathy.

## Treatment

A full screen for other sexually transmitted diseases should be encouraged. Partner notification is essential since such a high proportion of contacts will become infected. All sexual partners up to the previous three months should be traced and examined for evidence of infestation. All infected partners should be concurrently treated if possible. Patients should be advised to avoid close body contact until treatment, follow up checks and the partner notification and treatment are completed.

For eradication of the lice, lotions are more effective than shampoos and should be applied to all body hair. A second application within one week may be required. The treatment options are:

- malathion 0.5%. Apply to dry hair and wash off after 12 hours or
- carbaryl 0.5%. Apply to dry hair and wash off after two hours (not licensed for pubic lice in the UK) or
- phenothrin 0.2%. Apply to dry hair and wash off after two hours or
- permethrin 1% cream. Apply to damp hair and wash off after 10 minutes.

An alternative treatment is to shave all affected areas which may still be an option in developing countries.

Patients should be examined after one week for clearance. Nits (eggs) may be adherent to hair for some time and may be removed by using a fine comb. For infestation of the eyelashes, permethrin 1% can be used but the eyes should be kept tightly closed during and for 10 minutes after application. The lotion may be applied with a cotton swab. A non-chemical alternative is to apply a greasy emollient such as Vaseline to the eyelashes. This is then wiped off with the nits. The process may need to be repeated on a number of occasions.

## ARTHROPOD (INSECT AND MITE) BITES

Insects (with six legs) and arachnids (mites and spiders with eight legs) are responsible for arthropod bites in man. The genitals are commonly bitten by blood-sucking insects. Insects may be trapped in underwear or may seek the warm humid conditions of the genital area. Insect bites present as itchy papular or vesicular lesions, often grouped or in a linear distribution. There are four different patterns of bite commonly seen:

- red papules, occasionally with a central punctum
- vesicles, often clustered
- urticarial reactions with wheals
- haemorrhagic lesions (really vicious insects!).

When scratched, lesions may become secondarily infected or eczematous.

Insects that are commonly involved in biting the genitals include bed bugs, scabies, lice and fleas. The most common arthropod-induced skin lesion in man is the flea bite. There are many species of fleas. Some have a preferred host but others will bite and suck the blood of any suitable available host, including humans. Fleas use humans solely for feeding, whilse other hosts such as furry mammals provide food and housing.

The following commonly encountered insects tend to give characteristic bite patterns:
- mosquito – papules, blisters or urticated lesions
- fleas – three lesions in a row
- bedbugs – three lesions in a row in the morning, may urticate.

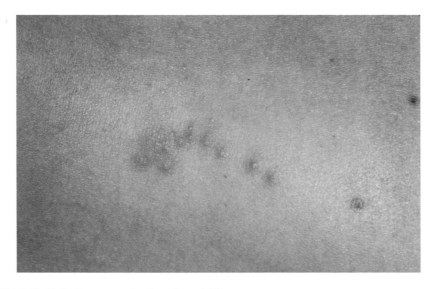

**FIGURE 3.7** Multiple linear papules from insect bites.

## KEY POINTS

⟩ Genital itching may be due to a skin disorder, localised infection or infestation or psychological causes.

⟩ Scabies is characterised by intense itch, especially at night.

⟩ The itching from pubic lice infestation occurs within a week of exposure.

⟩ Insect bites are most often characterised by itchy papules, usually in a linear distribution.

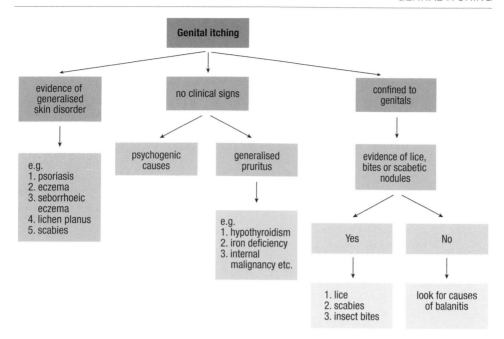

**FIGURE 3.8** Flow chart for diagnosing common causes of genital itching.

## CASE STUDY

Mike, a 22-year-old labourer, had suffered severe itching around his genital area for six weeks. The itching was spreading to the rest of his body and was particularly bad at night. He described the itching as 'the worse ever'. His doctor had tried various emollients and topical steroids with only limited benefit.

On arriving at the dermatology clinic it was noted that Mike was covered in scratch marks. Mike admitted that he did not currently have a girlfriend but 'slept around' by his own admission. There were no obvious burrows of scabies. However, there were small red papules on the glans penis and the shaft of the penis consistent with scabies infestation. He was treated for scabies but was advised to consult the genito-urinary medicine department for further sexually transmitted disease screening and partner notification.

# 4

# Problems with the foreskin

The function of the foreskin is to protect the glans penis. However, on occasions it may become diseased. Symptoms relating to foreskin dysfunction include:

- tightness and problems with retraction (phimosis)
- splitting of the foreskin, especially on intercourse
- persistent soreness or pain
- discharge or dribbling from the end of the foreskin.

## PHIMOSIS

Phimosis is a clinical sign and not a diagnosis. It may be a normal finding in boys but usually signifies a specific disease in men. There are various causes which are listed below:

- lichen sclerosus (common)
- lichen planus (common)
- sexually transmitted disease (common)
- hydradenitis suppurativa (rare)
- Crohn's disease (rare).

Men may experience a variety of other problems associated with the foreskin. A long foreskin is prone to cause symptoms of dribbling (*see* Chapter 1). Vigorous sexual intercourse may cause splitting of the foreskin, especially at the frenulum. Poor personal hygiene may lead to persistent soreness and inflammation of the foreskin and may result in balanitis (*see* Chapter 6). Failure to retract the foreskin regularly and to clean the glans penis will result in retention of smegma and the development of secondary infection (leading to infective balanitis). This may result in a penile discharge, especially in older men with poor hygiene.

### Diseases affecting the foreskin

1. Lichen sclerosus (also known as BXO).
2. All forms of balanitis (*see* Chapter 6).
3. Normal variants causing problems (*see* Chapter 1).
4. Zoon's balanitis (*see* Chapter 6).
5. Sexually transmitted diseases, e.g. gonorrhoea (*see* Chapter 9).

## LICHEN SCLEROSUS

Lichen sclerosus is also known by other names: lichen sclerosus et atrophicus and balanitis xerotica obliterans (BXO). The disease is now commonly known by the shorter term lichen sclerosus since atrophy is not always present. It is a chronic inflammatory dermatosis, mainly affecting the genitalia. Untreated, the disease often progresses to scarring.

### Incidence

Lichen sclerosus is around five times more common in women than men. The true

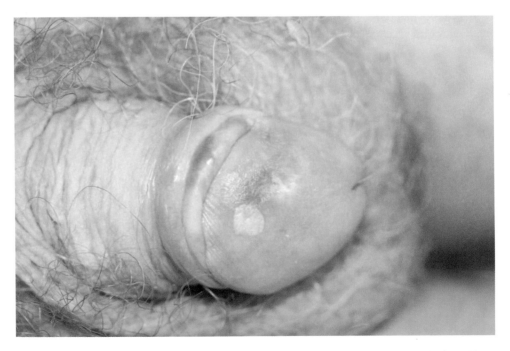

**FIGURE 4.1** Active lichen sclerosus of the penis with swelling and inflammation of the foreskin, pallor of the glans and active inflammation of the glans. The white plaque on the glans also represents lichen sclerosus (it was biopsied to exclude malignancy – *see* Chapter 5).

incidence in men is unknown and many may have been treated by circumcision during childhood. The disease is usually seen in uncircumcised men.

## Clinical history and examination

There are a large number of symptoms that may be associated with lichen sclerosus. Men often present with symptoms of phimosis. Retracting the foreskin may be difficult due to scarring or adhesions. Discomfort such as pain, soreness, bleeding, splitting of the foreskin and itching may occur, especially during or after sexual intercourse. Where scarring is a prominent feature (particularly around the urethral meatus) the symptoms may be related to micturition problems such as urinary retention, poor stream and dysuria.

Clinically, lesions may present as white, porcelain-like plaques on the glans penis or foreskin where scarring is present. Active inflammation is seen as red patches or plaques sometimes with purpura. Rarely, ulceration or bullae may be visible. Disease affecting the external urinary meatus may result in severe urethral stricture.

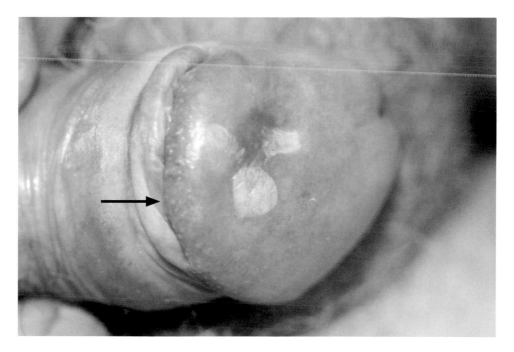

**FIGURE 4.2** Close up view of Figure 4.1. The foreskin has been pulled back to reveal pearly penile papules (arrow) around the corona.

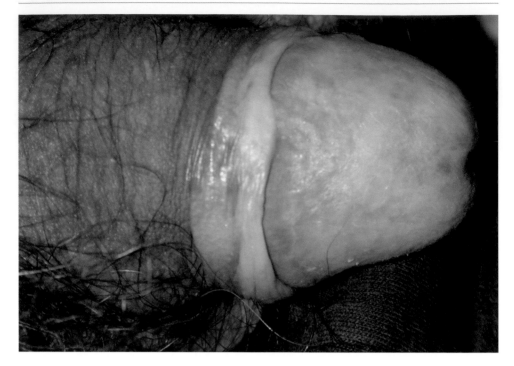

**FIGURE 4.3** Inactive lichen sclerosus showing typical pallor of the glans penis and prepuce.

## Diagnosis

Many cases of lichen sclerosus can be diagnosed clinically. However, co-existing disease such as Zoon's balanitis or infective balanitis is not uncommon and this may complicate diagnosis. Where doubt exists a skin biopsy should be taken. There is a characteristic histological appearance.

## Treatment

There are both medical and surgical treatments for lichen sclerosus. In most cases ultrapotent topical steroids (used under close specialist supervision) will improve symptoms. Even phimosis may respond to this therapy. There is little evidence for the efficacy of topical testosterone in males. Symptomatic phimosis and urethral stricture should be treated surgically and referral to a urologist is necessary. It is possible for lichen sclerosus to recur in a surgical scar following circumcision.

## Risk of penile cancer

Various studies have put the long-term risk of the development of squamous cell carcinoma of the penis in patients with lichen sclerosus at between 2 and 9% (*see*

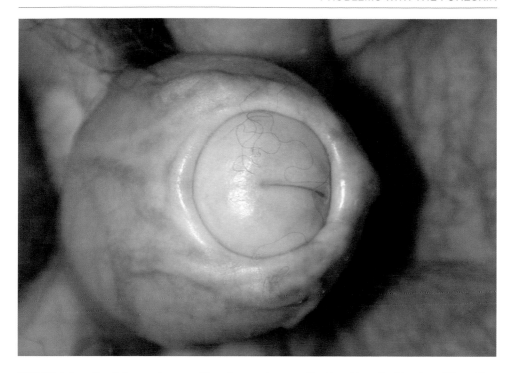

FIGURE 4.4 Inactive lichen sclerosus. The disease has resulted in phimosis. Atrophy of the skin of the prepuce makes the veins appear prominent.

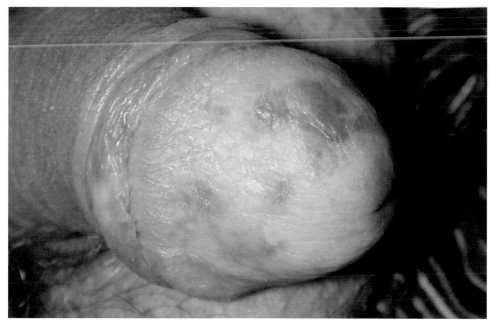

FIGURE 4.5 Lichen sclerosus of the glans penis showing active areas of inflammation (red) and pallor of the glans.

squamous cell carcinoma: Chapter 5, page 60). It is not known whether medical treatment of the disease reduces the risk of skin cancer, although it would seem prudent to follow up patients on a long-term basis.

## BALANITIS

Balanitis is dealt with in more detail in Chapter 6. However, it is important to understand why balanitis results in diseases of the foreskin. Balanitis refers to inflammation of the glans penis. When the foreskin is also involved this is termed balanoposthitis. The most common complication of balanoposthitis is phimosis.

## NORMAL VARIANTS CAUSING PROBLEMS

Occasionally a long foreskin will predispose towards problems. The commonest of these are trauma (e.g. being caught in a trouser zipper) and inflammation. Having a long foreskin may lead to problems with hygiene.

## ZOON'S BALANITIS (PLASMA CELL BALANITIS)

This rare inflammatory disorder is discussed in detail in Chapter 6 (page 66). It is usually a disease of both the glans penis and the foreskin and is extremely rare in circumcised males.

## SEXUALLY TRANSMITTED DISEASES AFFECTING THE FORESKIN

The common sexually transmitted diseases are dealt with in Chapter 9.

## KEY POINTS

> Phimosis is a sign and not a diagnosis. Causes should be sought.
> Lichen sclerosus in men requires specialised management.
> Untreated lichen sclerosus may lead to scarring and possibly penile cancer.
> Penile skin biopsy is often necessary to diagnose inflammatory dermatoses.

**CASE STUDY**

Philip was just 11 years of age when he realised his foreskin was very tight. Over the years he had experienced increasing problems retracting his foreskin. Now at the age of 30, the foreskin was so tight that it caused him pain on sexual intercourse and as a result his marriage was suffering. His general practitioner noted a phimosis and referred him to the local urology department where a circumcision was duly carried out. Unfortunately, within four weeks of the operation he developed an intensely sore red area around the scar. He was referred urgently to the dermatology department where a clinical diagnosis of lichen sclerosus was made. His symptoms responded within three weeks to ultrapotent topical steroids. He remained symptom-free during 12 months follow up.

# 5

# Lumps and lesions

Lesions on the genitals, the groins and the pubic area are very common. For the purposes of this book they are divided into a) benign lesions and b) pre-malignant and malignant lesions. The vast majority of genital lesions are benign. Some may be sexually acquired (e.g. viral warts, mollusca) and some may be part of a generalised condition (e.g. lichen planus). However, most occur as isolated skin lesions that happen to present in the genital area.

**TABLE 5.1** Genital skin lesions and normal variants

| | Common: Benign | See also | Rare: Benign |
|---|---|---|---|
| 1. | Basal cell papillomata (seborrhoeic warts) | Below | Angiokeratoma corporis diffusum (Anderson-Fabry disease) |
| 2. | Epidermoid cysts | Below | Keloids |
| 3. | Naevi | Below | Rare: Malignant and Pre-malignant Lesions |
| 4. | Dermatofibroma | Below | Bowenoid papulosis |
| 5. | Viral warts | Below | Bowenoid papulosis |
| 6. | Molluscum contagiosum | Chapter 10, page 113 | Bowen's disease |
| 7. | Angiokeratoma of Fordyce | Below | Squamous cell carcinoma |
| 8. | Skin tags | Below | Extra-mammary Paget's disease |
| 9. | Pearly penile papules | Chapter 1, page 3 | |
| 10. | Sebaceous hyperplasia | Chapter 1, page 4 | |
| 11. | Lichen planus | Chapter 6, page 69 | |
| 12. | Scabies | Chapter 3, page 28 | |

## COMMON BENIGN LESIONS

### 1. BASAL CELL PAPILLOMA (SYN. SEBORRHOEIC WART, SEBBORHOEIC KERATOSIS, SQUAMOUS PAPILLOMA)

This is the commonest benign skin lesion. They tend to asymptomatic but may occasionally itch. Lesions are usually pigmented and are more common in older people. They are relatively uncommon in black people. They range in size from 1mm to several centimetres and may be pedunculated. They can be found on the penis, in the groins and the pubic area but are relatively rare around the anal area. Lesions found at the anal margin resembling basal cell papillomata may need to be biopsied to exclude viral warts or Bowenoid papulosis (*see* page 56). On the penis, thighs and groins lesions are easily treated by simple curettage.

### 2. EPIDERMOID CYSTS (SYN. 'SEBACEOUS' CYST)

A common, asymptomatic lesion, particularly common on the scrotum. They are most often seen in the third and fourth decades of life. Milia are tiny epidermoid cysts. The skin overlying cysts may be pigmented, especially in people with dark skins. A central puctum is characteristic. They may occasionally become infected or calcify. They may be confused with giant mollusca (*see* molluscum contagiosum, page 52). It is not unusual for patients to have pricked and squeezed lesions, releasing their malodorous cheese-like contents (degraded keratin).

Treatment is rarely necessary. Incision and drainage results in a high recurrence rate, but excision of lesions is usually curative.

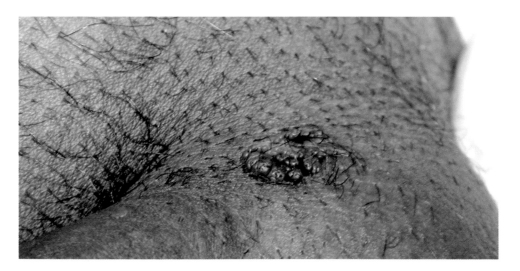

**FIGURE 5.1** Typical genital basal cell papilloma with warty surface.

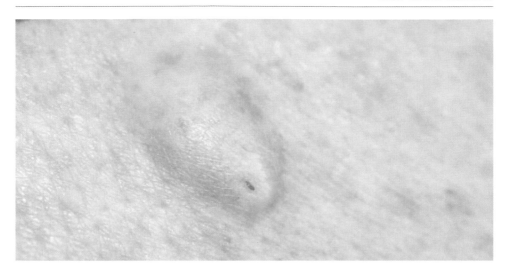

**FIGURE 5.2** Epidermoid cyst with central punctum.

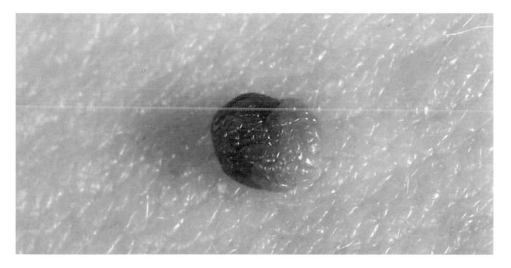

**FIGURE 5.3** Small 'warty' naevus.

## 3. NAEVI

Melanocytic naevi may be found anywhere on the skin including the genitals. Warty naevi (benign intradermal naevi) may occasionally be confused with basal cell papillomata, viral warts or even Bowenoid papulosis.

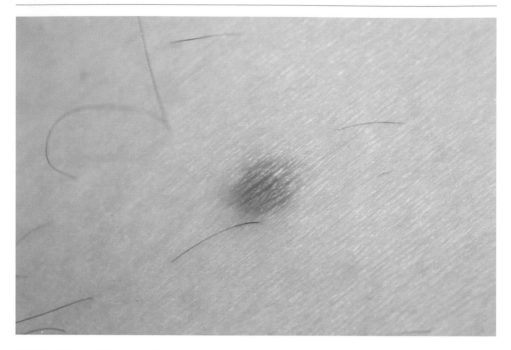

**FIGURE 5.4** Typical Dermatofibroma with pigmented overlying skin.

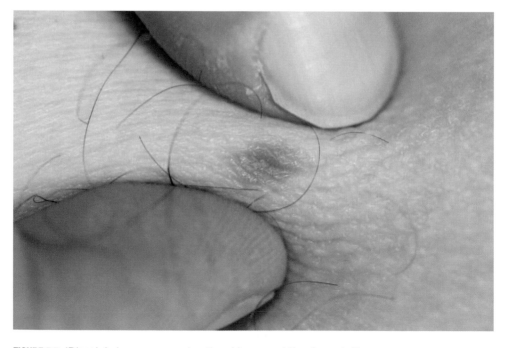

**FIGURE 5.5** 'Dimple' sign on squeezing the skin around the dermatofibroma.

## 4. DERMATOFIBROMA (HISTIOCYTOMA)

These common benign lesions are often found in the pubic area or on the thighs. They are relatively rare on the genitals themselves. Mostly they are asymptomatic but occasionally they may itch or become tender. Most lesions present in early adulthood as isolated dermal nodules measuring 5–10mm in diameter. The diagnosis is made clinically. The overlying skin is usually pigmented and when the nodule is laterally compressed it exhibits a characteristic 'dimple' sign due to tethering of the lesion to the overlying epidermis.

## 5. VIRAL WARTS

Genital warts are the commonest diagnosed viral infection in the UK and many other countries in the world. Infections are due to the human papilloma virus (HPV) of which over 70 subtypes have been identified. HPV types may be divided into low risk or high risk types depending on their association with pre-malignant and malignant diseases. Most genital HPV infections (over 90%) are due to the low risk types HPV 6 and 11. However, oncogenic types such as HPV 16, 18, 31 and 35 are associated with conditions such as Bowenoid papulosis (*see* page 56), penile intraepithelial carcinoma (*see* page 58) and penile squamous cell carcinoma (*see* page 60).

### Incidence

There has been a large increase in cases of genital warts over the last two decades. The majority of cases present in younger age groups: 20–24 years for men and 16–19 years in women. A large proportion of cases may remain silent

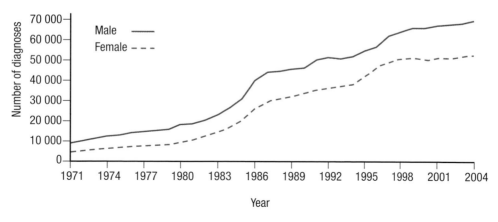

**FIGURE 5.6** Number of diagnoses of genital warts in genito-urinary medicine clinics in England and Wales 1971–2004.

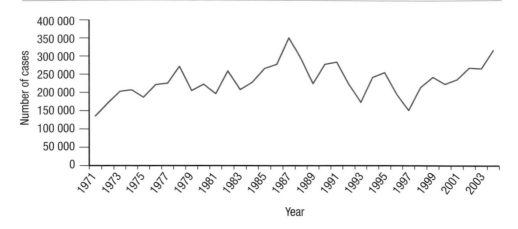

**FIGURE 5.7** Estimated cases of genital warts in the US based on visits to private physicians 1971–2004.

or asymptomatic. The lifetime risk for acquiring HPV infection sexually has been estimated to be around 80%. There are over 70 000 new cases of genital warts diagnosed yearly in the UK. The US has experienced a fourfold increase in prevalence over the last two decades. US data is estimated based on visits to private physicians. The relative standard error for the estimated US data (below) is between 20–30%.

## Clinical history and examination

HPV is spread by direct inoculation into the skin through microabrasions. There is then a latency period of months to years before clinical lesions become apparent. Genital warts appear as painless epidermal lesions. They may be plane (flat), filiform (fingerlike), papillomatous (small lumps), verrucous (warty) or pigmented. Most lesions are asymptomatic but rarely there may be itching or irritation. Common sites for presentation in men are the frenulum, the corona and glans penis, scrotal skin, the groin area and the perianal skin. It is also important to examine the urethral meatus where tiny mucosal lesions may present.

## Diagnosis

Diagnosis is made clinically but the wide range of clinical presentations may occasionally make diagnosis difficult. Use of topical 5% acetic acid is sometimes used by some physicians to highlight areas of HPV infection on the skin. Skin biopsy may be necessary where the diagnosis is uncertain. It is important not to confuse genital warts with the normal variant of pearly penile papules (*see* Chapter 1, page 3).

## Management

Around 20% of patients with genital warts have co-infection with other sexually transmitted diseases. All patients should be offered screening. Clinical examination of partners should also be offered and patients should be advised on safe sexual practice. The use of condoms significantly reduces the risk of acquiring genital warts.

Patients should be warned that there is no treatment modality that will prevent recurrences and treatment may have to be prolonged. A 'no treatment option' should be discussed since lesions are treated mainly for aesthetic reasons. Unfortunately, even with adequate therapy recurrence rates of over 50% at 12 months have been reported.

Therapy may be performed in the setting of a clinic or at home as a self-treatment, which tends to be popular.

### Self-treatment

Self-treatment includes the following:

1. Podophyllotoxin (a purified extract of podophyllin). Available in cream or liquid form. Applied to warts twice a day for three days and then no treatment for four days. The cycle can be repeated for up to six weeks depending on response.
2. Imiquimod 5% cream. A topical immuno-modulatory agent. Applied for three consecutive nights per week. The cycle can be repeated for up to 16 weeks.

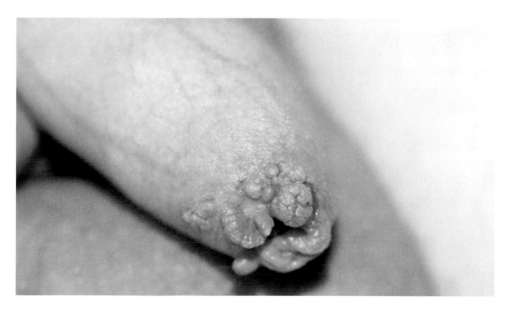

**FIGURE 5.8** Penile warts.

*Clinic-based treatment*

Most clinic-based therapies rely on local destruction of viral warts. They are often painful and have more side effects than home-based treatments.

1. Cryotherapy (liquid nitrogen or nitrous oxide).
2. Electrocautery or hyfrecation.
3. Surgery (curettage of lesions).
4. $CO_2$ Laser ablation.
5. Topical therapy
   - Trichloroacetic acid
   - Podophyllin
   - 5-fluorouacil
   - Salicylic acid.

## 6. MOLLUSCUM CONTAGIOSUM

Molluscum contagiosum is a viral infection that may present on the genitals. As with scabies, most cases are spread by non-sexual contact. However, when lesions arise on the genitals alone, the probability is that they are sexually transmitted. The virus is the molluscum contagiosum virus (MCV) which is a large DNA virus belonging to the molluscipox genus. Giant lesions may occur in patients with HIV and the presence of lesions may reflect immune deficiency (*see* Chapter 10,

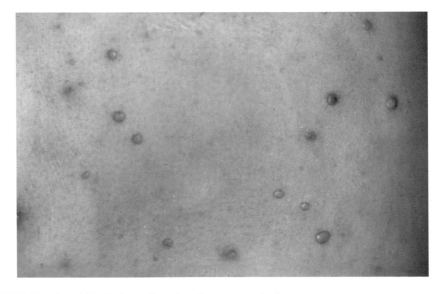

**FIGURE 5.9** Small umbilicated papules of molluscum contagiosum.

page 107). No accurate data exists on incidence of sexually acquired molluscum contagiosum.

## Clinical history and examination

The condition commonly presents as a sexually transmitted infection on the genitals in the 20–29 year age group. The incubation period is from 14 days to six months. Lesions are asymptomatic unless they become inflamed or secondarily infected.

Lesions may be between 1 and 10mm in diameter. They appear as umbilicated, hemispherical pearly papules and may be isolated or occur in groups of 10–20 lesions.

## Diagnosis and treatment

The condition is usually diagnosed clinically. When in doubt a biopsy can be taken which demonstrates typical histopathological findings. Lesions spontaneously resolve in three to six months without treatment. Destruction of lesions and the production of an inflammatory reaction may accelerate resolution. Various therapies have been tried including cryotherapy, curettage, diathermy and laser ablation. Tradition methods include puncturing lesions with a sharp instrument dipped in 80% phenol. More recently there is evidence imiquimod cream 5% may be useful as well as 1% hydrogen peroxide cream. Lesions may heal with scarring whether or not they have been treated.

## 7. ANGIOKERATOMA OF FORDYCE

These small vascular, asymptomatic papules measuring 1–5mm in diameter, are commonly found on the genitals. They are made up of capillaries and may occasionally bleed. They are more common in white males and the scrotum is a favoured site. The lesions occur in all ages but are more common in the elderly. They require no treatment but will often respond to hyfrecation, cautery or laser. The differential diagnosis is that of Anderson-Fabry disease (*see* below).

## 8. SKIN TAGS (ACHROCHODON)

Skin tags are common pedunculated protrusions, most often existing in the groins and other flexures. They are usually small, measuring around 2–4mm but may be up to several centimetres with an elongated stalk. They often co-exist with basal cell papillomata. If necessary, they can be treated by cautery or cryotherapy.

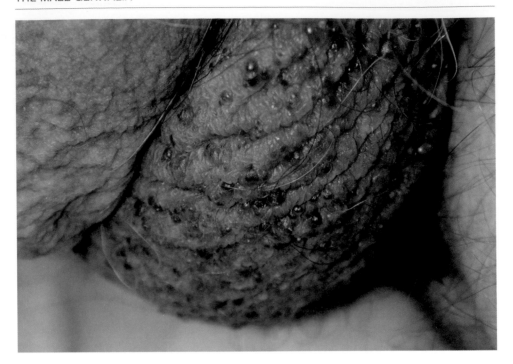

**FIGURE 5.10** Scrotal haemangiomas.

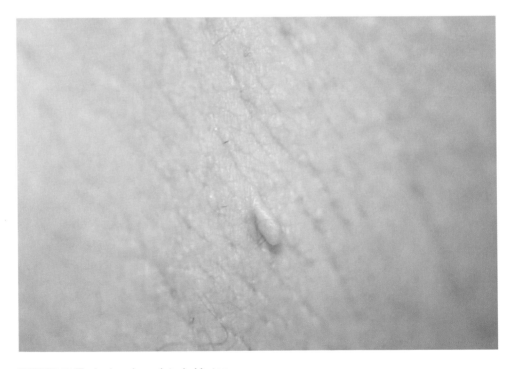

**FIGURE 5.11** Typical pedunculated skin tag.

## 9. PEARLY PENILE PAPULES (*see* Chapter 1, page 3)

## 10. SEBACEOUS HYPERPLASIA (*see* Chapter 1, page 4)

## COMMON NORMAL VARIANTS

## 1. LICHEN PLANUS (*see* Chapter 6, page 69)

## RARE BENIGN LESIONS

## 1. ANGIOKERATOMA CORPORIS DIFFUSUM (ANDERSON-FABRY DISEASE)

As the name suggests this condition is characterised by multiple angiokeratomas, particularly seen on the thighs and in the groin area. It is a rare (around 1:40 000 population) X-linked multi-system disorder and therefore only seen in males. It is an important differential diagnosis when vascular lesions are seen on the skin, since the condition is treatable.

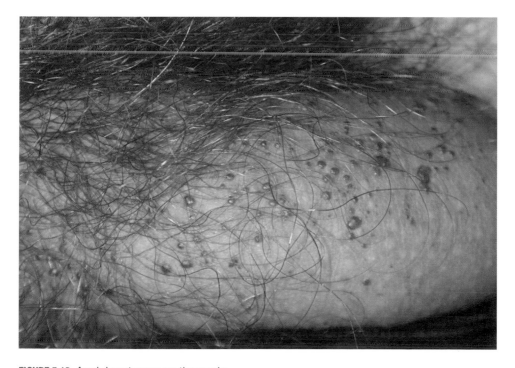

**FIGURE 5.12** Angiokeratomas on the penis.

## 2. KELOIDS

Keloids are hypertrophic scars rarely seen on the genitals. They represent an overgrowth of fibrous tissue. They are more commonly seen in black people and usually present between 10 and 30 years of life.

## PRE-MALIGNANT AND MALIGNANT LESIONS

## 1. BOWENOID PAPULOSIS

Bowenoid papulosis is a papular eruption of the genitals seen in both sexes, thought to be caused by infection with human papilloma virus (HPV). It may be considered as an epidermal cellular atypia somewhere in the spectrum between viral warts and Bowen's disease (*see* below). As such, it has a (low) malignant potential. Although a number of HPV subtypes are linked to Bowenoid papulosis, the strongest link is with HPV 16.

### Incidence

This condition affects both sexes equally. There is a strong association with genital warts and the disease is primarily seen in young sexually active adults. All races are affected.

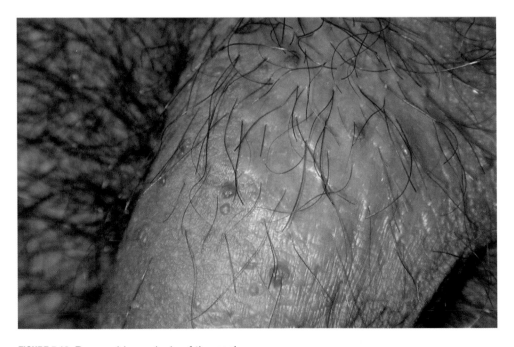

**FIGURE 5.13** Bowenoid papulosis of the penis.

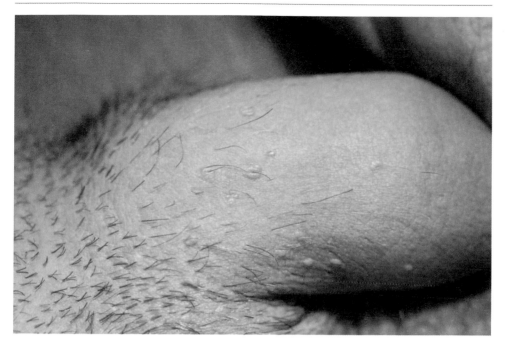

**FIGURE 5.14** Bowenoid papulosis. These lesions could easily be mistaken for plane warts.

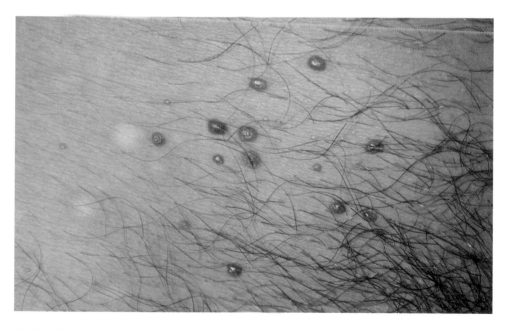

**FIGURE 5.15** Bowenoid papulosis affecting the lower abdomen. Note the hypopigmented areas resulting from previous treatment with cryosurgery.

## Clinical history and examination

Lesions are usually asymptomatic, multiple, may resemble viral warts and may occur anywhere on the genitals and surrounding skin. They are pigmented, flat-topped papules, varying from red to dark brown. Occasionally, they may fuse to form larger plaques.

## Diagnosis

The differential diagnosis lies between genital warts, benign warty lesions such as basal cell papillomas and forms of intraepithelial neoplasia (*see* Bowen's disease below).

## Treatment

Treatment is necessary since there is a low risk of malignant change (unknown but probably less than 2%) and a theoretical risk of transmission of HPV to sexual partners. Barrier methods of contraception should be used while lesions are present and partners should be screened for sexually transmitted disease and have cervical smears performed.

A number of treatment options have been documented although the evidence for efficacy is lacking in most. Cryosurgery is usually successful as is curettage and cautery, although there is a recurrence rate. Topical agents such as imiquimod, trichloro-acetic acid and 5-fluouracil cream may be used but are usually highly irritant.

## 2. BOWEN'S DISEASE/ERYTHROPLASIA OF QUEYRAT

Bowen's disease of the penis, Erythroplasia of Queyrat (EQ) and Bowenoid papulosis are all forms of intraepithelial carcinoma. The nomenclature is poor and other terms such as penile intraepithelial neoplasia are also used. The term Bowen's disease is used to describe intraepithelial neoplasia at any body site, whereas EQ is a term specific to the penis.

## Incidence

Rare with few reports in the literature. Most cases appear around 50 years of age.

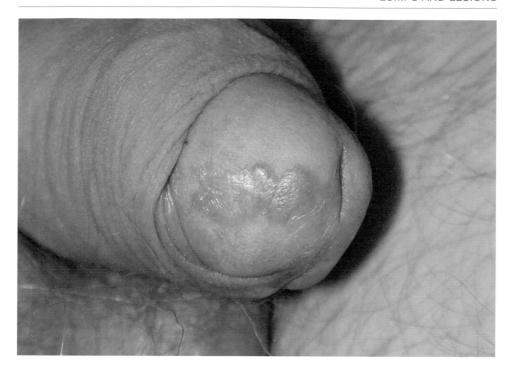

**FIGURE 5.16** Localised area of penile intraepithelial neoplasia.

## Clinical history and examination

The condition presents mainly on the glans in uncircumcised men. The range of presentations can be large and the diagnosis may be missed if the condition is not considered. Patients may present with redness of the glans penis, bleeding, penile pain, itching, ulceration, urinary symptoms and foreskin problems. The clinical findings are often non-specific with the clinical picture ranging from isolated papules or plaques on the penis to verrucous lesions.

## Diagnosis

A high index of suspicion is most likely to lead to a biopsy and hence accurate diagnosis. Any patient who has a persistent penile problem (such as a chronic lesion), especially those not responsive to appropriate topical therapies, should have a skin biopsy to exclude malignant and pre-malignant processes.

## Treatment

Treatment is specialised. The condition is rare and patients should be referred to a local specialist in this area. Various therapies have been employed including use of 5-fluouracil cream, carbon dioxide laser ablation, photodynamic therapy and cryotherapy. Wherever possible surgical excision (including Moh's micrographic surgery) will give a good histological specimen that can be examined for completeness of excision.

## 3. SQUAMOUS CELL CARCINOMA OF THE PENIS

Squamous cell carcinoma of the penis is a rare but serious cancer with a high mortality. Late presentation and mis-diagnosis account for some of this mortality. There are clear risk factors including smoking and contact with carcinogens such as oils, tar and arsenic. There is a link with human papilloma virus and the condition may be a rare, late complication of photochemotherapy for treatment of psoriasis. Chronic inflammation is also a risk factor and this is particularly seen in untreated lichen sclerosus. The condition is extremely rare in circumcised men. Phimosis is present in a high percentage of men with the disease.

### Incidence

Penile cancer is rare with around 100 deaths per year in the UK. It accounts for around 0.5% of malignancies in Western countries. It is much more common in under-developed countries where co-existing infections such as HIV are an aetiological factor and may account for as much as 20–30% of all cancers in men.

### Clinical history and examination

Symptoms such as itch, pain, bleeding and irritation may have been present for many months or years. Men often complain that they have had problems with the foreskin for some time before seeking attention.

Penile cancers are most commonly found on the glans penis (around 50%) and the prepuce (around 20%). In addition, tumours may involve both the glans and the prepuce together. Lesions tend to present as small nodules, non-healing areas or ulcers. Phimosis may make examination difficult. There may be co-existing signs of inflammatory conditions such as lichen sclerosus.

Penile cancer metastases first to the inguinal lymph nodes. Palpable lymphadenopathy may be present if this occurs. Untreated, the disease is fatal within two years in the majority of cases.

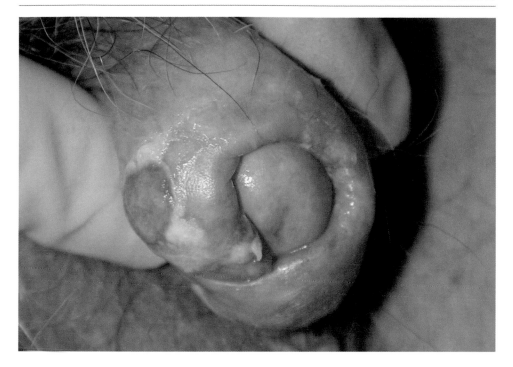

**FIGURE 5.17** Squamous cell carcinoma of the prepuce.

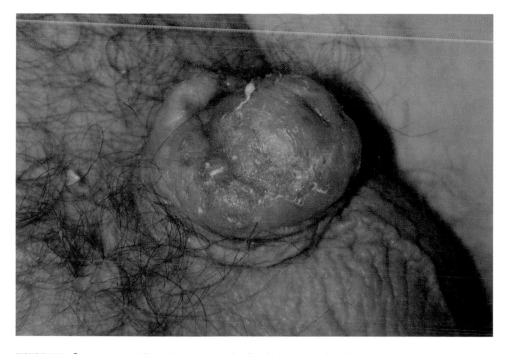

**FIGURE 5.18** Squamous cell carcinoma developing in longstanding lichen sclerosus.

## Diagnosis

Although the cancer is rare, a high level of suspicion is needed for any penile lesion that is ulcerated, non-healing, bleeding or has been present for a long time. The diagnosis is confirmed by biopsy. Occasionally multiple biopsies may be necessary. If clinically suspicious, a lesion should be fully excised even if initial histological analysis fails to confirm cancer.

## Treatment

Treatment of penile cancer is the remit of the specialised urologist and referral to a specialist regional centre is necessary once the diagnosis is confirmed. Complete resection of the tumour is the treatment of choice and this may lead to penile amputation. Both radiotherapy and chemotherapy have been used for metastatic disease.

## 11. EXTRA-MAMMARY PAGET'S DISEASE (*see* Chapter 2, page 19)

## KEY POINTS

> Most genital lesions are benign, asymptomatic incidental findings.
> Common skin lesions often occur on the genitals.
> Viral lesions such as warts and molluscum are usually sexually transmitted.
> Persistent lesions may rarely represent malignant or pre-malignant conditions.
> When in doubt of diagnosis a biopsy is necessary.

## CASE STUDY

Harold had just celebrated his 74th birthday when he noticed an unpleasant discharge coming from his penis. He had not had sex for 11 years since the death of his wife and thought nothing of it. After four months he noticed blood on his underwear and consulted his general practitioner. Harold had not retracted his foreskin for several years and having the foreskin pulled back caused him a great deal of pain. His general practitioner noted a large friable fleshy nodule on the glans penis. He went first to the dermatology clinic where a biopsy confirmed the clinical suspicion of squamous cell carcinoma. He had a limited resection of the penis under the care of the urologists. Sadly, he developed inguinal lymph node swelling two months later and subsequently died of metastatic carcinoma.

# 6

# The red glans penis

The red glans penis is a common clinical problem, especially in uncircumcised men. The term *balanitis* is used to describe inflammation of the glans penis whilst *balanoposthitis* refers to inflammation of both the glans and the foreskin. Balanitis is a symptom, not a diagnosis, and causes for penile inflammation should be sought. Perhaps the most common problem is poor personal hygiene. This predisposes to irritation and infection under the foreskin. This may result in phimosis or a penile discharge. In the dermatology clinic the commonest causes of balanitis are inflammatory dermatoses. Sexual health physicians may see more cases of infective balanitis.

The main causes of balanitis are listed below:

|  | Diagnosis | See also |
|---|---|---|
| **Inflammatory dermatoses** | Eczema-allergic contact | Chapter 11 |
|  | Eczema-irritant contact | Chapter 11 |
|  | Eczema-seborrhoeic | Chapter 11 |
|  | Psoriasis | Chapter 11 |
|  | Zoon's balanitis | *See* below |
|  | Lichen planus | *See* below |
|  | Lichen sclerosus | Chapter 4 |
|  | Reiter's syndrome | *See* below |
| **Infective** | Infective balanitis | Below and Chapter 2 (candidosis) and Chapter 9 |
| **Other** | Drug related | *See* below |

Patients with balanitis may complain of penile discharge, dysuria (*see* also Chapter 9), soreness and inability to retract the foreskin. Patients may also be aware of an unpleasant smell. Clinically, it may be very difficult to distinguish between various forms of balanitis since they often present in similar ways with a non-specific redness of the glans.

## ZOON'S BALANITIS (PLASMA CELL BALANITIS)

This rare form of balanitis was described in 1952. The aetiology is unknown but it has been postulated that the condition may represent a chronic irritant mucositis.

### Incidence

Zoon's balanitis occurs mainly in middle-aged and older men. It is almost exclusively a disease of uncircumcised men. The incidence is unknown but of over 250 consecutive men presenting to our male genital dermatosis clinic, 9% were diagnosed with Zoon's balanitis.

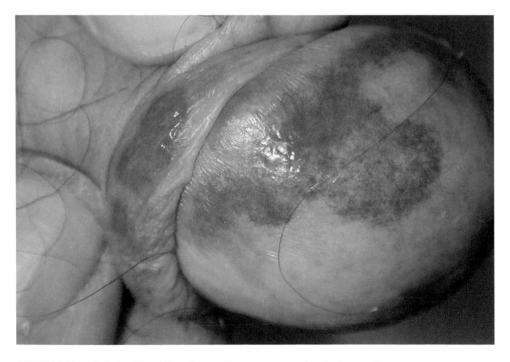

**FIGURE 6.1** Zoon's balanitis of the glans with a corresponding lesion on the prepuce.

## Clinical history and examination

Many patients may be unaware of symptoms. Staining of underclothes with blood and discharge may be an incidental finding. Occasionally soreness and itching may occur but presentation most often comes about after the patient notices the red appearance of the glans penis.

Solitary, shiny or glistening erythematous plaques may be seen on the glans penis. There is often a corresponding lesion on the prepuce resembling an ink blot pattern. Lesions may have a 'cayenne pepper' appearance due to pinpoint purpura.

## Diagnosis

Diagnosis may be confused with other forms of balanitis, such as fixed drug eruptions, erosive lichen planus (*see* below), psoriasis, seborrhoeic eczema and pre-malignant lesions such as Erythroplasia of Queryat (*see* Chapter 5, page 58). Skin biopsy is usually necessary to confirm diagnosis. A dense dermal infiltrate of plasma cells on histology is characteristic. Secondary infection is very common in these patients and microbiological swabs may demonstrate growths of anaerobic bacteria, coliforms and streptococci.

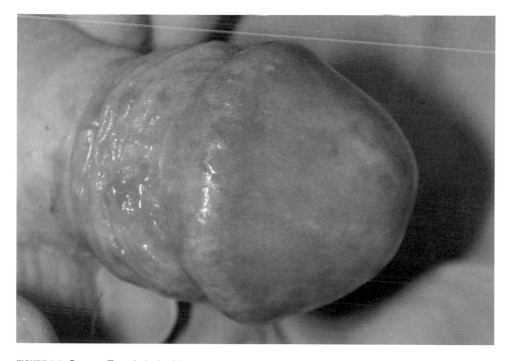

**FIGURE 6.2** Severe Zoon's balanitis.

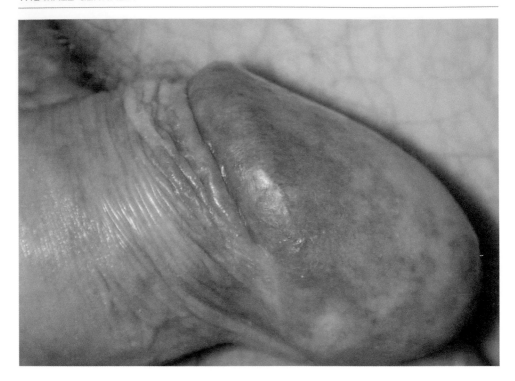

**FIGURE 6.3** Zoon's balanitis of the glans and prepuce.

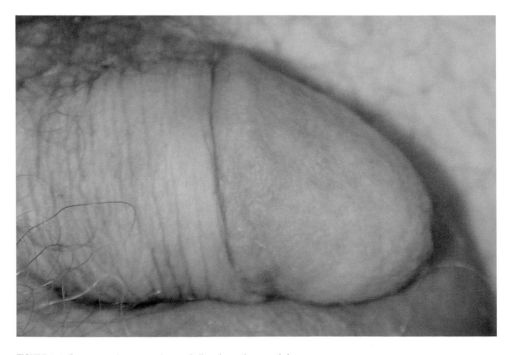

**FIGURE 6.4** Same patient as above following circumcision.

## Treatment

Zoon's balanitis may be very resistant to treatment. Topical agents are standard first-line therapy. Corticosteroids, antibacterial agents and antifungal agents have all been used with some success. Occasionally, patients respond to hygiene measures alone, particularly if their previous level of hygiene was poor. The definitive treatment is circumcision which is almost always curative. The $CO_2$ laser has also been used with some success.

# LICHEN PLANUS

Lichen planus is a common inflammatory dermatosis of unknown aetiology. The disease commonly affects the genitals as part of a generalised eruption but may also affect the genitalia alone. It may become chronic in nature but the majority of cases resolve within 12 to 18 months. Lichenoid (lichen planus-like) drug eruptions may occur on the penis (*see* below).

## Incidence

Lichen planus can occur at any age. It affects males and females equally and all racial groups.

## Clinical history and examination

On the penis burning and intense itching are common. Sexual intercourse may be uncomfortable. Men are often alarmed by the red appearance of the glans penis. When the rash affects other body sites it tends to be extremely itchy.

Classically, the eruption is symmetrical and itchy. It may affect any area of skin but particularly involves the flexor aspects of the wrists, the nails and mucous membranes. Lesions are characteristically small, flat-topped red-purple papules. They have a lacy or fern-like scale called Wickham's striae. Lesions on the glans penis in uncircumcised men may appear as often non-specific erythematous plaques.

There is a rare erosive form of the disease which is extremely uncommon in men and affects mucosal surfaces. Resolving lichen planus may give rise to post-inflammatory hyperpigmentation which may persist for many months.

## Diagnosis

The diagnosis is usually made clinically. Lichen planus of the penis may be the only presentation of the disease on the body. Single, isolated lesions may

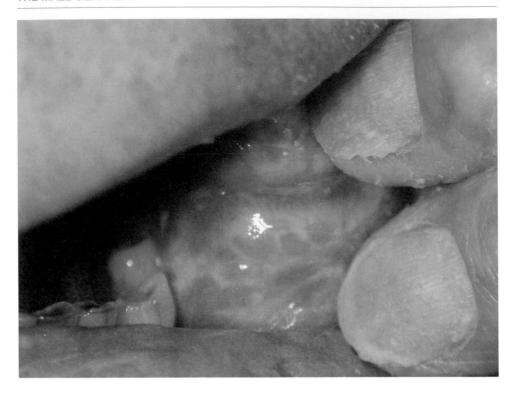

**FIGURE 6.5** Lichen planus of the nails (pitting) and the oral mucosa (Wickham's striae).

resemble Erythroplasia of Queyrat. Skin biopsy may be helpful where diagnosis is uncertain or where the condition has failed to respond to appropriate therapy. The differential diagnosis includes most of the inflammatory dermatoses affecting the penis but also pre-malignant lesions.

## Treatment

The treatment of choice is the use of potent or ultrapotent topical steroids, under close supervision. Washing the skin with a soap substitute will reduce irritation. There is some evidence that cessation of smoking may be beneficial in penile lichen planus. Circumcision, particularly for erosive lichen planus has a role in some patients. Systemic steroids are sometimes necessary for severe or erosive forms of the disease.

## Lichenoid drug eruptions

There are a number of drugs that can give rise to a lichen planus-like eruption

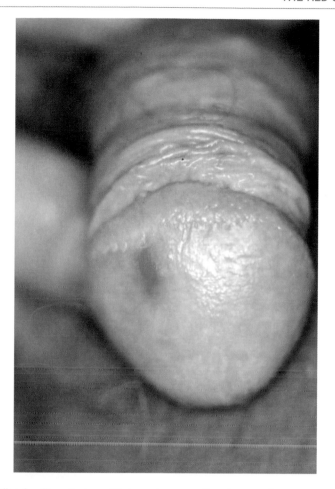

**FIGURE 6.6** Localised solitary lesion of lichen planus on the glans penis.

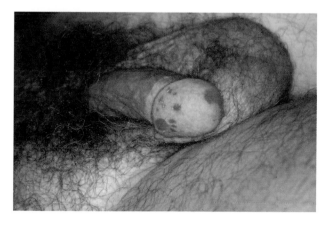

**FIGURE 6.7** Multiple lesions of lichen planus on the glans penis.

on the skin. Whilst they tend to cause a widespread lichenoid eruption the rash may occasionally be localised just to the genitals. The eruption may be clinically identical to lichen planus and may occur several months after commencing the offending drug. There are a large number of drugs that have been reported to cause a lichen planus-like eruption. These include:

- aciclovir
- antimalarials
- betablockers including metoprolol and propranolol
- captopril
- carbamazapine
- ethambutol
- gold salts
- interferon
- methyldopa
- phenothiazines
- temazepam
- tetracyclines
- thiazide diuretics.

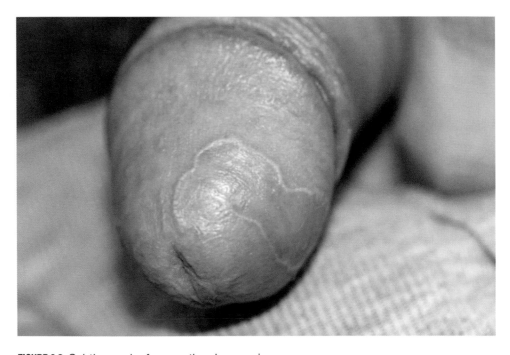

**FIGURE 6.8** Subtle annular form on the glans penis.

## REITER'S SYNDROME

Reiter's syndrome is normally defined as a triad of urethritis, arthritis and conjunctivitis. It is an important disease in men with genital symptoms since it may present with skin lesions and may be caused by a sexually transmitted disease (most commonly chlamydia). The disease can also arise as a result of gastro-intestinal infections. The disease tends to present in young men. It is the commonest cause of arthritis in men aged between 20 and 40 years.

There is a strong association with the HLA B-27 antigen and an association with HIV has also been identified. The usual presentation is with an oligoarthritis, most often of the knee, around three weeks after an episode of urethritis or diarrhoea.

Skin, oral and penile lesions may occur. Keratoderma blenorrhagica consists of hyperkeratotic nodules on the feet which may be indistinguishable from pustular psoriasis. It may also occur on the extensor aspects of the legs, the dorsae of the toes and on the fingers, nails and hands. The rash is often widespread and appears around four to eight weeks after the onset of arthritis. Painless vesicles and erosions with an erythematous base may affect the oral mucosa.

Penile lesions occur in approximately a quarter of patients. In uncircumcised men the glans develops erythematous, moist erosions. These may easily be mistaken for psoriasis (see Figure 11.3, page 122). As these coalesce the characteristic sign of circinate balanitis is seen. In circumcised men the erosions become crusty and scaly and may appear similar to the keratoderma lesions elsewhere on the body.

Reiter's syndrome may be confused with psoriasis. Patients should be screened for sexually transmitted disease including HIV. The disease resolves spontaneously in two-thirds of patients within six months.

## INFECTIVE BALANITIS

Poor hygiene is often a pre-disposing factor to infective balanitis. Causes of this form of balanitis may be divided into non-sexual infections and sexually transmitted diseases.

### a. Non-sexually transmitted infections

There are a number of organisms that commonly cause balanitis. Candida is a common cause, especially in patients with diabetes (see also Chapter 2, page 14). Other organisms that may become pathogenic include anaerobes, group B streptococci and coliforms.

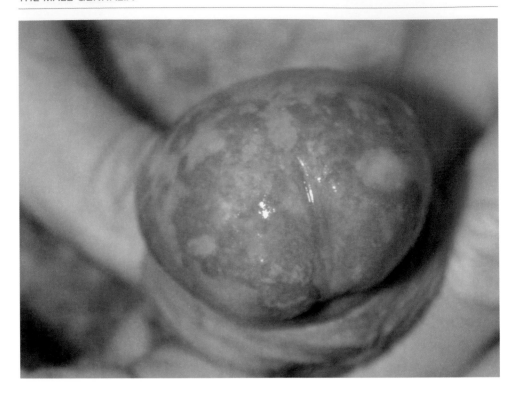

**FIGURE 6.9** Candida balanitis.

## b. Sexually acquired infective causes of balanitis

These include gonorrhoea (*see* Chapter 9), trichomonal species, syphilis and herpes simplex (*see* Chapter 8, pages 83–93). Organisms such as gardnerella vaginalis that may cause penile discharge and dysuria can also cause infective balanitis (*see* Chapter 9).

## DRUG-RELATED BALANITIS

There are two important forms of drug eruption that may affect the genitals. Lichenoid drug eruptions affecting the penis have been discussed above. Fixed drug eruptions are relatively uncommon but often affect the genitals.

Fixed drug eruption tends to occur on the extremities, the face and the genitals. The eruption is characterised by well-demarcated erythematous plaques that recur at the same site or sites each time the offending drug is used. There may be a central blister in the middle of lesions occasionally confusing it with erythema multiforme.

Drugs that have been implicated in fixed drug eruption are listed below:

- amoxicillin
- barbiturates
- chlordiazepoxide
- dapsone
- oxyphenylbutazone
- paracetamol
- phenolphthalein
- propranolol
- quinine
- salicylates
- sulphonamides
- tetracyclines.

## KEY POINTS

❱ There are many causes of a red glans penis including inflammatory dermatoses and infections.

❱ Investigation including microbiological swabs and skin biopsy are often necessary to diagnose the red glans penis.

❱ Taking a good history is essential, particularly asking about past and present skin disease and current and previous medication.

---

**CASE STUDY**

Graeme, 66, had not had sex for three years due to an unsightly and sore rash on his glans penis. After finding a new partner he decided to seek help. His foreskin was difficult to retract and the glans penis was moist, fiery red in places with a yellowish discharge. The rash improved markedly with an antibiotic-steroid cream but recurred quickly on cessation. A diagnosis of Zoon's balanitis was made at the local dermatology clinic. He eventually ended up having a circumcision which cured the rash.

# 7

# Problems with pigmentation

The male genitals are normally more pigmented than other areas of skin. This is particularly noticeable in the pigmentation of the scrotum. The contrast between the skin colour of the genitals and the rest of the body is more striking in people with dark skin. There are a number of normal variants in pigmentation that have been discussed in Chapter 1.

Common disorders of pigmentation discussed in this chapter:
1. Hyperpigmentation problems:
   - drug causes
   - as part of a generalised pigmentary problem, e.g. Addison's disease
   - post-inflammatory hyperpigmentation
   - genetic disorders (the majority have lentiginous hyperplasia).
2. Hypopigmentation problems:
   - vitiligo
   - scarring conditions, e.g. lichen sclerosus (*see* Chapter 4, page 38)
   - post-inflammatory hypopigmentation.
3. Normal variants (*see* also Chapter 1):
   - median raphe
   - penile melanosis.

## 1. HYPERPIGMENTATION PROBLEMS

Genital pigmentation may be isolated or may be a part of a widespread pigmentation disorder. Systemic disorders such as Addison's disease will give hyperpigmentation over various parts of the body, not just the genitals. Drugs may cause a generalised hyperpigmentation or the pigmentation may occasionally be localised to the genitals alone.

**TABLE 7.1** Causes and conditions associated with excess genital pigmentation

| Common causes | See also | Rare causes | See also |
|---|---|---|---|
| Median raphe | Chapter 1, page 5 | Drugs | Fixed drug eruption Chapter 6, page 74 |
| Post-inflammatory hyperpigmentation | Chapter 11 | Addison's disease | |
| Penile melanosis | Normal variants (below) | Lentiginous hyperplasia | |

## Drug causes of genital pigmentation

A number of drugs known to cause skin pigmentation may cause genital pigmentation, including:

- amiodarone
- antimalarial drugs
- tetracyclines
- phenothiazine
- phenytoin
- rifampicin
- topical hydroquinones
- AZT.

**FIGURE 7.1** A localised area of post-inflammatory hyperpigmentation with a small area of active eczema above it.

## Causes of post-inflammatory hyperpigmentation

Post-inflammatory hyperpigmentation is more common in patients with pigmented skin. It may occur after most causes of acute skin inflammation, e.g.

- post-surgical
- resolving lichen planus
- resolving eczema
- fixed drug eruption
- post-infectious, e.g. recurrent herpes simplex.

## Lentiginous hyperplasia

A lentigo (*plural lentigines*) is a melanocytic lesion of the skin clinically similar to a freckle. Lentigines on the genitals and mucosal surfaces may indicate a genetic disorder. There are a number of familial lentiginoses that affect the genitalia including Peutz-Jegher's syndrome, Laugier-Hunziker syndrome, Carney complex (includes LAMB and NAME syndromes) and LEOPARD syndrome. The presence of genital freckling should alert the clinician to the possibility of a genetic problem. Specialist genetic or dermatological advice should be sought.

## 2. HYPOPIGMENTATION PROBLEMS

There are a number of common causes of white skin on the genitals. The majority of these are due to post-inflammatory hypopigmentation. Pale or white skin may arise as a result of melanin loss (post-inflammatory hypopigmentation, vitiligo), reduction in blood flow (e.g. due to vasoconstriction arising from topical steroid use, topical local anaesthetics) and scarring (e.g. lichen sclerosus).

**TABLE 7.2** Causes and conditions associated with pale and white areas on the genitals

| Common causes | See also | Rare causes | See also |
|---|---|---|---|
| Vitiligo | Below | Syphilis | Chapter 8, page 83 |
| Lichen sclerosus | Chapter 4, page 38 | Paget's disease | |
| Post-inflammatory hypopigmentation | *See* below | Mycosis fungoides | |
| Viral warts | Chapter 5, page 49 | Penile striae (due to topical steroid use) | |
| Median raphe | Chapter 1, page 5 | | |

## Vitiligo

Vitiligo is a common skin condition resulting in destruction of melanocytes. It occurs in all races at a rate of 1–2%. It commonly presents between 10 and

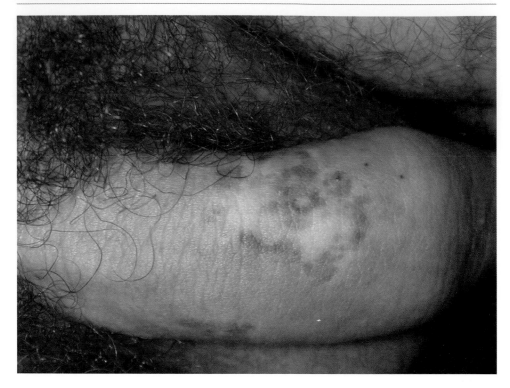

**FIGURE 7.2** Vitiligo of the shaft of the penis. The surrounding area of hyperpigmentation is not uncommon. The differential diagnosis is penile melanosis (*see* below).

30 years of age. The genitals are often affected and may be the only site involved. The condition is thought to be due to an autoimmune process and as such may be related to other autoimmune conditions such as thyroid disease.

Diagnosis is made clinically but may be facilitated by the use of the Wood's light in order to visualise areas of pigment loss. Treatment options on the genitals are limited. Although photochemotherapy (PUVA), topical steroids and topical immunomodulatory agents have been successfully used for vitiligo on other areas of the body, they are relatively contra-indicated on the genitals. PUVA is carcinogenic and the topical agents run the risk of reactivating dormant viral conditions (herpes simplex virus, human papilloma virus).

## Post-inflammatory hypopigmentation

Post-inflammatory hypopigmentation is more common than hyperpigmentation and can similarly be as a result of acute inflammation in the skin. The causes include:

- post-operative, e.g. after cryosurgery (common after treatment for viral warts)

- eczema
- lichen planus
- post herpes simplex infection
- lichen sclerosus.

## 3. NORMAL VARIANTS

There are some normal variants that may present as a pigmentary problem. The median raphe may be hyperpigmented or hypopigmented. The genitals are normally pigmented in relation to surrounding skin and this is often more obvious in men with pigmented skins.

Penile melanosis is a descriptive term used to describe a condition where the penile skin is irregularly pigmented. This is a benign condition distinct to post-inflammatory hyperpigmentation. It would appear that the skin is both hyperpigmented and hypopigmented. There may be some confusion with lentiginous hyperplasia (*see* above).

## KEY POINTS

- Both hyper- and hypopigmentation may follow a resolving skin disorder.
- Drugs may cause genital pigmentation.
- Genital pigmentation may be a part of a generalised disorder such as a genetic or metabolic condition.
- Vitiligo and lichen sclerosus are common causes of a reduction in genital pigmentation.

## CASE STUDY

A 23-year-old man who refused to give his name arrived at the genito-urinary clinic complaining of pale patches on his penis. He had heard this could be a presentation of syphilis and was worried. No infectious cause was found and he was referred to the dermatology clinic. Under the ultraviolet light a number of depigmented areas of skin were identified on the penis, the thighs and back. Because of his pale skin these areas were not readily visible under normal light. A diagnosis of vitiligo was made but despite a number of therapeutic measures no improvement occurred.

# 8

# Genital ulcers and blisters

There are a large number of causes of genital erosions and ulcers, which often develop following the formation of a blister. Any blistering condition may result in genital ulcers. This includes generalised blistering disorders such as bullous pemphigoid, pemphigus and erythema multiforme and localised blistering diseases such as herpes simplex and herpes zoster infection. Causes of genital ulcers, erosions and blisters may be divided into infectious and non-infectious types:

**TABLE 8.1** Causes of genital erosions, blisters and ulcers

|  | Common | Rare |
|---|---|---|
| **Sexually transmitted infections** | Syphilis (below) | |
| | Herpes simplex virus (below) | |
| | | Lymphogranuloma venereum (below) |
| | | Chancroid (below) |
| **Other causes** | Trauma | Fixed drug eruption (*see* Chapter 6) |
| | Candida | |
| | Bacterial infection, e.g. staphylococcus, streptococcus | Bullous disease, e.g. pemphigus, pemphigoid |
| | Inflammatory bowel disease (Ulcerative colitis, Crohn's disease) | Behcet's disease (below) |
| | Lichen sclerosus (*see* Chapter 4) | Erosive lichen planus (*see* Chapter 6) |
| | Erythema multiforme | Squamous cell carcinoma (*see* Chapter 5) |

## SYPHILIS

Syphilis is due to infection with the organism Treponema pallidum. This is a motile, regularly close-coiled spirochaete. It is an unusual organism in that it can not be cultured in the laboratory, although it may be observed *in vitro* using dark-field microscopy or fluorescent staining. The organism can only be identified in the primary and secondary stages of syphilis. Both of these forms of the disease are highly infectious.

## Epidemiology

The prevalence of syphilis is increasing in Europe and the USA. There has been a sharp increase in incidence from 1995 to date (*see* below). The UK has seen a 1500% increase in reports of syphilis diagnosed in genito-urinary medicine clinics between 1995 and 2004. The highest rates appear to be in homosexual men. In the developing world the prevalence of syphilis remains high.

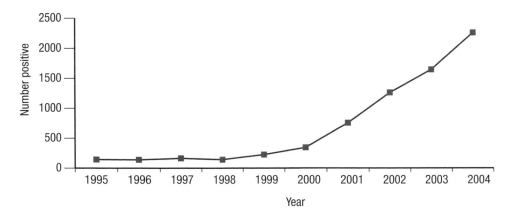

**FIGURE 8.1** New diagnoses of syphilis in the UK 1995–2004.

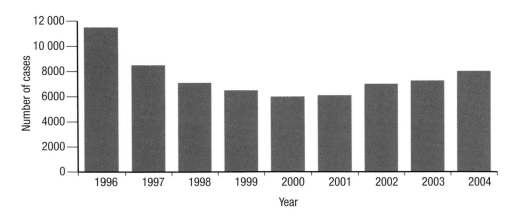

**FIGURE 8.2** Cases of primary and secondary syphilis reported in the US 1996–2004.

## Classification of acquired syphilis

- Early infectious stages: primary syphilis and secondary syphilis.
- Late latent (after two years).
- Late syphilis – tertiary syphilis (gummatous, cardiovascular, neurosyphilis).

## Clinical history and examination

### 1. Primary syphilis

There are often no symptoms. The most consistent finding of primary syphilis is the genital chancre (ulcer). A painless papule appears at the site of inoculation between 9 and 21 days (range 9–90 days) after exposure. This is usually single and painless. Within several days the papule ulcerates. The ulcer measures 1–2cm in diameter and has a clear base without exudate. Oro-genital sex is a major risk factor for transmission of the infection and primary lesions may be found on the lips, tongue, pharynx and tonsils. Homosexual men may be unaware of the primary lesion if it is situated in the anus. The regional lymph nodes may be enlarged but are usually non-tender.

The main differential diagnosis of primary syphilis is that of herpes simplex. The following table outlines the main features of each:

**TABLE 8.2**

|  | Herpes simplex | Primary syphilis |
| --- | --- | --- |
| History | Prodromal itching or burning | No prodromal symptoms |
| Examination | Multiple painful vesicles<br>Non-indurated thin border | Usually single non tender lesion<br>Firm, indurated border |
| Regional lymph nodes | Enlarged and tender | Enlarged, non-tender |
| Sexually active patient | Yes | Yes |
| Outcome | Chronic, relapsing | Curable with treatment |

### 2. Secondary syphilis

The onset of secondary syphilis may range from six weeks to six months after initial infection and the primary chancre may still be present when secondary lesions occur. There may be constitutional symptoms such as fever, headache, myalgia, malaise, arthritis and hepatitis which can precede a generalised rash. The rash may present in a number of forms (the 'syphilides'), but it usually is a polymorphic, symmetrical eruption that tends to also affect the palms and soles. The skin is itchy in around 40% of patients. The other manifestations of secondary syphilis are:

- generalised painless lymphadenopathy (75% inguinal and 60% generalised)
- oro-genital mucosal lesions (30% mucous patches and snail track ulcers)

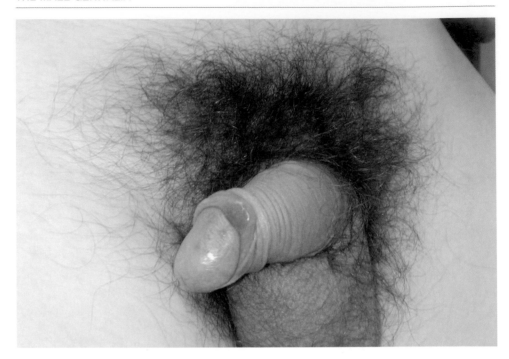

**FIGURE 8.3** Primary syphilis: chancre on penis.

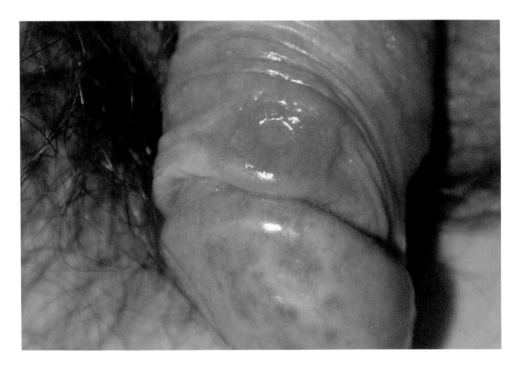

**FIGURE 8.4** Chancre: close up.

- hepatomegaly (10% usually sub-clinical)
- patchy 'moth eaten' hair loss
- condylomata lata (warty papules and plaques in the perianal area)
- anterior uveitis and optic neuritis.

## Diagnosis of syphilis

The diagnosis may be made by dark-field microscopic examination of a smear taken from a chancre or lesion of secondary syphilis or from a lymph node aspirate. Serological testing of blood is necessary. A number of serological tests are currently available:

- reaginic (cardiolipin-based) tests: Venereal Disease Research Laboratory test (VDRL) and rapid plasma reagin test (RPR)
- specific treponemal tests: T. pallidum haemagluttination assay (TPHA), micro-haemagluttination assay for T. pallidum (MHA-TP), T. pallidum particle agluttination test (TPPA), fluorescent treponemal antibody absorption test (FTA-abs test), treponemal enzyme immunoassay (EIA)/ IgG, IgG immunoblot test for T. pallidum
- specific anti-T. pallidum IgM antibody tests.

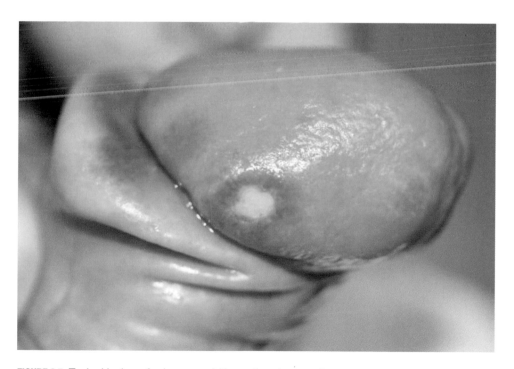

FIGURE 8.5 Typical lesion of primary syphilis on the glans penis.

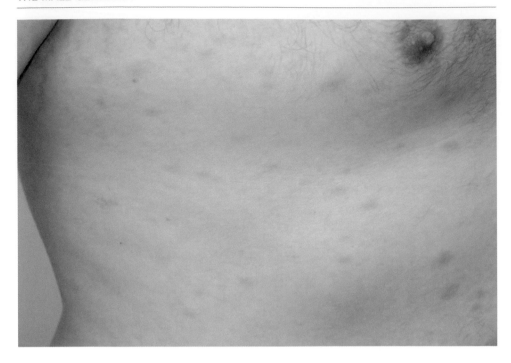

**FIGURE 8.6** Symmetrical rash of secondary syphilis.

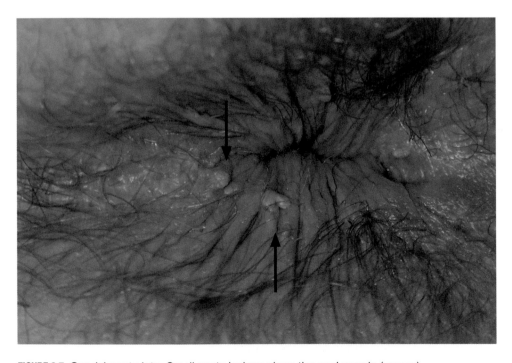

**FIGURE 8.7** Condylomata lata. Small warty lesions along the anal margin (arrows).

Preliminary screening tests:

- EIA/ IgG-test
- TPHA, MHA-TP or TPPA may be used (VDRL or RPR are also occasionally used in addition)
- FTA-abs test or EIA-IgM test may be the first test to be positive if primary syphilis is suspected.

Confirmatory tests if initial screening is positive (always repeat positive tests to confirm results):

- Treponemal EIA, FTA-abs test
- IgG immunoblot test for T. pallidum if it is suspected TPHA/ MHA-TP and/ or FTA-abs test results are false positives.

## Treatment

As with all sexually transmitted diseases, partner tracing and treatment is essential. All partners within the previous six months should be traced and monthly serological tests should be performed for three months. Screening for concomitant infections (particularly HIV) is necessary.

Penicillin remains the treatment of choice:

- procaine penicillin G 600–750mg daily intramuscularly for 10 days or
- benzathine benzyl penicillin, 2.4 Million Units intra-muscular stat single dose (US) or twice one week apart (UK).

For penicillin allergic patients:

- doxycycline 100mg twice daily for two weeks or
- azithromycin 500mg daily for one week or
- tetracycline 500mg four times daily for two weeks or
- erythromycin 500mg four times daily for two weeks.

The patient should be warned of the possibility of a Jarisch-Herxheimer reaction that may occur on initiation of therapy. This involves fever and constitutional symptoms such as malaise, headache, myalgia and pyrexia. Anaphylaxis is a possibility and resuscitation equipment should be available following the initial dose.

## Follow up

Patients should be followed up to confirm cure and to detect relapse and re-infection. This is done clinically and serologically by checking VDRL and RPR for 6–12 months. It should be noted that specific treponemal tests will usually be positive for life.

As with all sexually transmitted infections, patients with early syphilis should be offered partner notification.

## HERPES SIMPLEX (HSV)

There are two types of herpes simplex virus: HSV 1 and HSV 2. Transmission of the virus is by close contact with an infected individual. The virus is inoculated into the skin through tiny breaks in the mucosal surface. The virus can invade and replicate in the nervous system and can lie dormant in nerve cell ganglia. Reactivation often occurs and may be precipitated by stress or trauma.

### Incidence

Herpes simplex occurs worldwide. Disseminated forms are more prevalent due to the increased incidence of HIV. Between 1971 and 2004 the number of cases of genital herpes simplex diagnosed in genito-urinary medicine clinics in England and Wales rose by 5 and 20 times in males and females respectively. In the United States estimated numbers of office visits for genital herpes increased fivefold between 1971 and 1994.

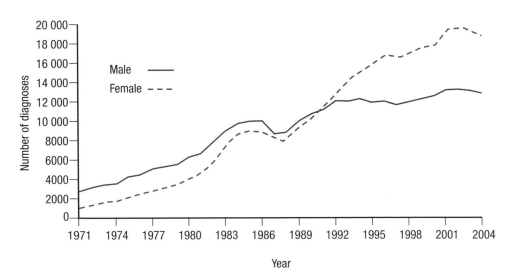

**FIGURE 8.8** Number of cases of genital herpes seen in genito-urinary clinics in England and Wales 1971–2004.

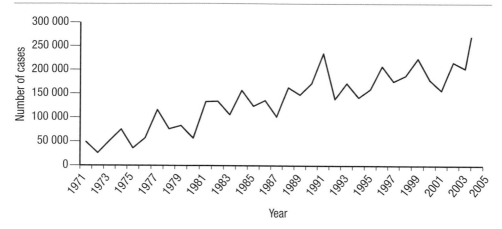

**FIGURE 8.9** Estimated cases of genital herpes in the US based on visits to private physicians 1971–2004.

## Clinical history and examination

Around 70% of infected individuals may be asymptomatic. The diagnosis may only come to light when their partner displays symptoms. Sexually acquired herpes simplex occurs on the genitals within 7 days of exposure. Prior to the development of lesions, prodromal symptoms such as fever, headache and myalgia or local soreness may be experienced. Small vesicles then occur, most commonly on the glans penis and/or the foreskin. These are around 2–3mm in diameter on an erythematous base. Lesions may also be found on the thighs and buttocks. The usual symptoms are of local soreness and pain. Urethritis occurs in approximately 40% of affected men. Healing, initially with crusting, takes place after around 5–15 days. The median period of viral shedding (infectious period) is 12 days. Healing may result in skin changes of post-inflammatory hypo- or hyper-pigmentation.

The major problem associated with herpes simplex infection is the high frequency of reactivation of the virus resulting in multiple recurrent episodes. Around 90% of patients with genital HSV 2 develop recurrences. The recurrent episodes tend to be similar to the initial one and may be precipitated by stress or sexual intercourse. Recurrent herpes infection causes significant physical and psychological morbidity. A number of patient support groups have been formed to help affected individuals (*see* Appendices).

## Diagnosis

Although the diagnosis is usually made clinically, it may be confirmed by culture or by polymerase chain reaction (PCR). A swab of the blister fluid can be sent

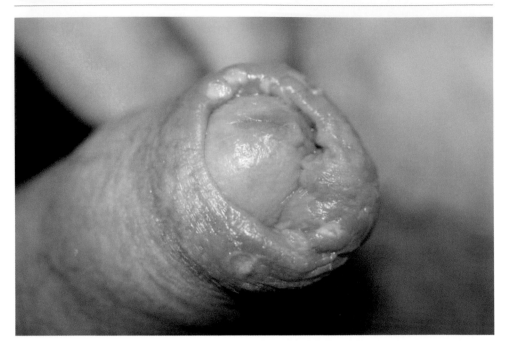

**FIGURE 8.10** Sloughy ulcers on the foreskin from HSV causing extreme soreness and swelling.

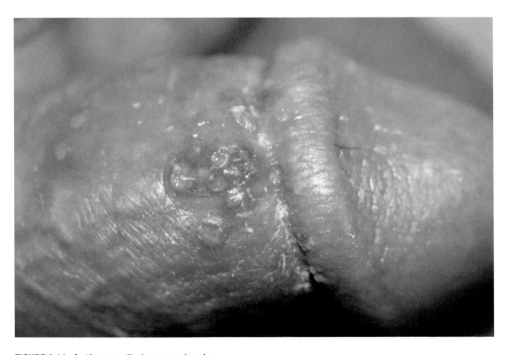

**FIGURE 8.11** Active penile herpes simplex.

for microbiological culture (the virus is isolated in tissue culture). The virus may also be detected using electron microscopy. For rapid diagnosis of HSV, PCR can be used to look for HSV DNA. This test has the added benefit of being able to detect asymptomatic viral shedding.

## Management

The skin often becomes extremely inflamed in HSV infection causing additional problems such as urinary retention, phimosis and secondary infection. Regular cleansing of the skin with antiseptics is beneficial as is the treatment of any secondary bacterial infection. There are a number of antiviral drugs available. It should be stressed to the patient that only the acute episode is being treated and recurrence is likely. Drugs currently in use:

- aciclovir 200mg five times daily for five days or
- famciclovir 250mg three times daily for five days or
- valaciclovir 500mg twice daily for five days.

The antiviral agents only reduce the virus shedding period by a short period. They do not prevent recurrences. For recurrent HSV infection, low dose antiviral therapy (e.g. aciclovir 200mg or 400mg twice daily) for a period of weeks or months may however be helpful. Psychological morbidity may require the intervention of specialist help.

## LYMPHOGRANULOMA VENEREUM

This sexually transmitted disease is caused by the bacterium chlamydia trachomatis. It is rare in the US and UK but is endemic in India and Southeast Asia, East and West Africa, South America and the Caribbean.

The disease has three stages:

- Stage One: small painless papules appear on the genitals which ulcerate and then disappear within a few days.
- Stage Two: the inguinal lymph glands swell within two to six weeks and become painful. Constitutional symptoms such as fever, malaise, pyrexia and muscle pain often occur.
- Stage Three: years after initial infection a chronic inflammatory process causes fistulae, abscesses, lymphatic damage, strictures and scarring of the genital, pelvic and perianal regions.

Diagnosis may be made by an antibody blood test or by demonstrating intracellular inclusion bodies in stained smears from active lesions. The disease is treated using any of the following antibiotic regimes:

- doxycycline 100mg twice daily for 21 days or
- erythromycin 500mg four times daily for 21 days or
- azithromycin 1g orally once weekly for four weeks.

## CHANCROID

Chancroid is a sexually transmitted disease due to the organism Haemophilus ducreyi. It is rare in the US and UK but relatively common in Africa, Asia and the Caribbean.

The disease is characterised by painful genital ulcers and painful inguinal lymphadenopathy (buboes). The initial lesion is of a small papule, pustule or vesicle on the genitals especially at sites of friction. It occurs within a week of exposure to the bacterium through sexual intercourse. Painful ulceration soon occurs. The inguinal lymph nodes become painful, enlarged and hard.

The disease is curable if treated early. Diagnosis may be made by culture but this is not available in most parts of the world. Where culture is unavailable diagnosis must be made clinically and appropriate therapy started. Several antibiotics are effective for treatment:

- azithromycin 1g orally as a single dose or
- ceftriaxone 250mg intramuscular single dose or
- erythromycin 500mg four times daily orally for seven days or
- ciprofloxacin 500mg twice daily orally for three days.

As with any genital ulcer disease the risk of HIV is higher in these patients. Screening for HIV, syphilis and other causes of genital ulceration is necessary.

## BEHCET'S DISEASE

Behcet's disease is a rare disease characterised by recurrent oral and genital ulceration and uveitis. The cause of this multi-system disease is unknown. It is rare in the UK and US (around five cases per 100000 population) but more frequent in the Middle and Far East and Mediterranean region (around 1 case per 10000 population).

Diagnostic criteria:

- recurrent oral ulceration.

Plus two of the following:

- recurrent genital ulceration

- uveitis
- skin lesions of erythema nodosum, pustular lesions or acne-like nodules
- positive pathergy test (the development of a pustule or indurated nodule at the site of a needle prick or injection of normal saline into the skin).

There are a number of other clinical manifestations that may occur. These include fever, malaise, arthralgia, sore throats and tonsillitis, anorexia, urethritis and psychiatric illness.

There are no diagnostic tests available. A range of therapies have been tried with limited success. For milder cases topical corticosteroids and antibiotic/antiseptic agents may help.

## KEY POINTS

❭ The incidence of genital herpes simplex and syphilis continues to rise in most countries.
❭ HSV and syphilis are the commonest causes of genital ulceration worldwide.
❭ Screening for concomitant infections such as HIV is important in all patients diagnosed with a sexually transmitted infection.
❭ A detailed sexual history is needed in patients presenting with genital ulceration.

---

**CASE STUDY**

A young homosexual man presented to the genito-urinary medicine clinic with a painless ulcer on his glans penis, present for one week. He admitted to having unprotected intercourse with multiple partners at a party two weeks previously. He had a 1cm ulcer on the lateral aspect of his glans penis and bilateral inguinal node swelling. A clinical diagnosis of primary syphilis was made and he was screened for other sexually transmitted diseases including HIV at his request. His tests confirmed primary syphilis and he was treated with intramuscular penicillin. Unfortunately, he failed to attend for follow up appointments.

# 9

# Penile discharge and dysuria

Urethral discharge in men is the typical presentation of urethritis. The term urethritis is usually reserved for sexually transmitted diseases. The diagnosis of urethritis is confirmed by taking a swab from the urethra and demonstrating the presence of pus. The usual symptoms are dysuria (discomfort on passing urine) and discomfort or irritation at the tip of the penis. Balanitis may also occur. Some men may be asymptomatic. Urethritis is divided into two groups: gonococcal and non-gonococcal urethritis (NGU).

The diagnosis of urethritis is important for a number of reasons:
- most cases are sexually transmitted
- the risk of acquiring and transmitting HIV is increased with urethritis
- the organisms responsible for most cases of urethritis in men are important causes of infertility in women
- urethritis can lead to problems such as sexually acquired arthritis, epididymitis and prostatitis.

There are causes of urethritis not related to sexually transmitted infections. These include post-traumatic urethritis (e.g. found in up to a fifth of men practising self-catheterisation), and a number of infectious syndromes such as Reiter's syndrome (*see* page 73).

For the purposes of this book we focus on the sexually acquired causes of urethritis: gonorrhoea and NGU.

## GONORRHOEA

Gonorrhoea is an infection of the mucous membrane surfaces caused by the bacterium Neisseria gonorrhoeae. The organism is a highly infectious gram negative diplococcus, commonly referred to as the gonococcus. A single act of unprotected sexual intercourse with an affected individual will give a transmission rate of between 30% and 70%. The risk of a woman developing gonorrhoea from a man is much higher than for a man developing the disease from an infected woman. In men, an acute purulent urethritis occurs in the majority of infected individuals, although some may be asymptomatic.

## Incidence

Gonococcal infections are approximately one and a half times more common in men. As with other sexually transmitted diseases the frequency is highest in adolescents and young adults. Gonorrhoea is a worldwide problem with around 200 million new cases every year. The UK has seen an increase of 111% between

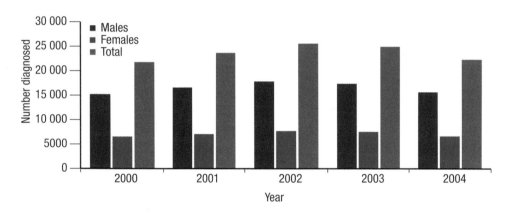

FIGURE 9.1 Cases of gonorrhoea in the UK 2000–2004.

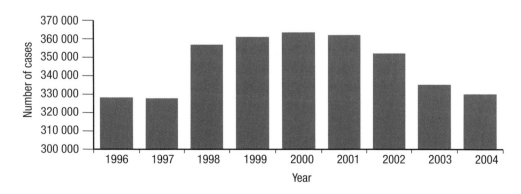

FIGURE 9.2 Cases of gonorrhoea in the US 1996–2004.

1995 and 2004. Some ethnic groups have a disproportionately high rate of gonorrhoea. In the US there are around 330 000 new cases each year reported but the true figure is probably considerably higher. The problem is more acute in underdeveloped parts of the world.

## Clinical history and examination

Symptoms of urethral discharge, discomfort and dysuria due to urethritis occur in most men with gonorrhoea, although the severity of these symptoms varies. If infection has reached the posterior urethra symptoms of painful erections, frequency of micturition and urgency may be experienced. The clinical examination reveals a purulent urethral discharge often with an inflamed urethral meatus.

Unilateral pain and swelling of the scrotum signifies epididymitis. Rectal infection is usually asymptomatic but pharyngeal infection gives soreness, discomfort and sometimes dysphagia. In 1–2% of cases a disseminated form of gonorrhoea occurs with joint pains, constitutional symptoms such as fever and disseminated pustules on the body.

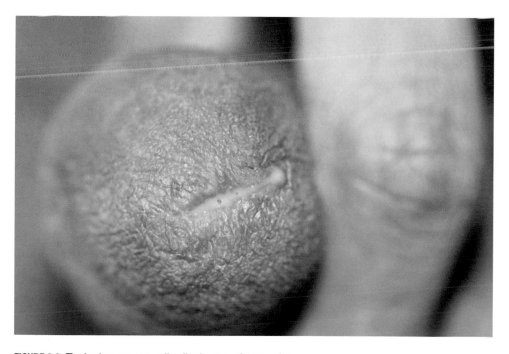

**FIGURE 9.3** Typical creamy penile discharge of gonorrhoea.

### Diagnosis

A urethral discharge may not be clinically evident and 'milking' or 'stripping' the penis may be necessary to obtain a suitable urethral specimen. A urethral swab should be taken from between 1 and 2cm into the urethra. A gram stain is a rapid, cheap and sensitive test. A gram stain showing five or more white blood cells per oil immersion field with intracellular gram negative diplococci has a specificity for gonorrhoea of over 95% (*see* Figure 9.4). Urine can be tested using nucleic acid amplification techniques to screen for gonorrhoea. The organism should also be cultured and antibiotic sensitivities established.

Swabs should be taken from all possible exposed sites such as the pharynx and rectum.

It is important to screen for other sexually transmitted infections, particularly syphilis and chlamydia trachomatis (*see* below).

### Management

A significant emerging problem with the treatment of gonorrhoea is antibiotic resistance. Penicillin, tetracycline and quinolone resistance is becoming common. Resistance varies according to geographical location, for example gonorrhoea

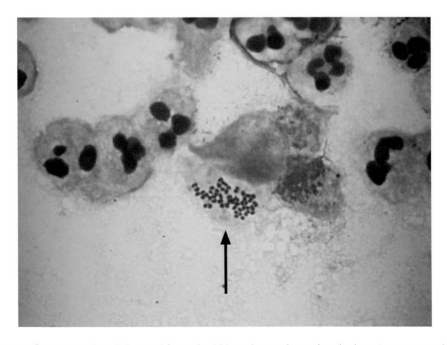

**FIGURE 9.4** Gram negative diplococci (arrow) within polymorphonuclear leukocytes seen under high power microscopy.

acquired in South East Asia should be presumed to be both penicillin and quinolone resistant.

There are a number of recommended treatment regimes for uncomplicated urethral gonorrhoea:

- ceftriaxone 250mg intramuscularly as a single dose or
- ciprofloxacin 500mg orally as a single dose or
- ofloxacin 400mg orally as a single dose or
- cefixime 400mg orally as a single dose or
- spectinomycin 2g intramuscularly as a single dose.

Penicillin may still be used where the isolate is known to be penicillin-sensitive, e.g. amoxicillin 2g or 3g orally with probenecid 1g orally as a single dose. Concomitant anti-chlamydial treatment, e.g. azithromycin 1g twice daily or doxycycline 100mg twice daily for seven days is recommended.

It is essential to perform a test of cure of all affected sites within seven days. Once again, partner notification with up to three months of look back period and test of cure is important.

It is very important to know the resistance of gonorrhoea locally. In addition, knowledge of foreign travel by affected patients is essential. The graph below demonstrates the wide range of differences in ciprofloxacin resistance gonococci between countries.

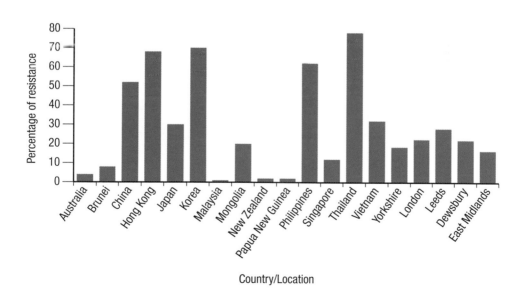

**FIGURE 9.5** Gonorrhoea and drug resistance 2002–2003.

## NON-GONOCOCCAL URETHRITIS (NGU)

Non-gonococcal urethritis is a general term for all the other causes of urethritis other than gonorrhoea. In many cases no organism is found and treatment has to be empirical.

There are a number of causes of NGU:

- chlamydia trachomatis 30–50% cases
- mycoplasma genitalium
- ureaplasma urealyticum
- herpes simplex virus
- *E. coli* (in homosexual men)
- no identifiable organism 20%
- Reiter's syndrome
- other rare causes.

### Incidence

The incidence of NGU in the United States is around three million new cases per year. There are tens of millions of new cases each year worldwide.

### Clinical history and examination

Patients with NGU have a longer incubation period compared with patients with gonorrhoea. Around a quarter of men with NGU are asymptomatic, although they may have a urethral discharge when examined. Typical symptoms experienced include urethral discharge and dysuria. It is rare for patients to experience systemic symptoms or urinary symptoms. As with gonorrhoea, there is often a creamy muco-purulent urethral discharge.

### Diagnosis

*1. If microscopy and investigation available*

Urethral culture is necessary to exclude gonorrhoea. Urine can be tested using nucleic acid amplification techniques to exclude both gonorrhoea and chlamydia. Demonstration of pus in the anterior urethra confirms a diagnosis of urethritis. Traditionally, patients have been diagnosed and treated according to the gram stain obtained from an endo-urethral swab inserted 1–2cm into the urethra. If gram negative intracellular diplococci are seen the patient is treated for gonorrhoea. If these organisms are not seen the patient is treated for NGU (*see* below).

## 2. If microscopy unavailable

If a muco-purulent discharge is demonstrated the patient should be treated for both gonorrhoea and NGU. A simple test to perform is the two-glass urine test. This consists of asking the patient to retract the foreskin and pass urine into two clean specimen glasses (10–20ml in the first and the rest into the second). If the urine is hazy 5% acetic acid is added until all phosphate crystals are dissolved. In the presence of pus in the anterior urethra, the haze will persist in the first glass due to pus cells, threads or flecks and the second glass will remain clear.

## Management

Recommended treatment regimes for NGU:
- doxycycline 100mg orally twice daily for seven days or
- azithromycin 1g orally as a single dose.

Alternative regimes:
- erythromycin 500mg orally four times daily for seven days or 500mg twice daily for 14 days or
- tetracycline 500mg orally four times a day for seven days or
- ofloxacin 200mg orally twice daily or 400mg daily for seven days.

Follow up should take place 7–14 days after the initial consultation.

## CHLAMYDIA

Since chlamydia trachomatis is responsible for up to half the cases of NGU, it is worth considering it in more detail.

## Incidence

Chlamydia is currently the commonest sexually transmitted infection in the UK diagnosed in genito-urinary medicine clinics with over 100000 cases in 2004. Between 1995 and 2004, the number of cases diagnosed in genito-urinary medicine departments increased by 221%. The highest rates of chlamydia in the UK are among 16–19-year-old females and 20–24-year-old males. There are around a million new reported cases of chlamydia in the US each year with an estimated 2.8 million Americans infected. Some figures suggest at-risk groups such as sexually active adolescent girls have an incidence of 10%.

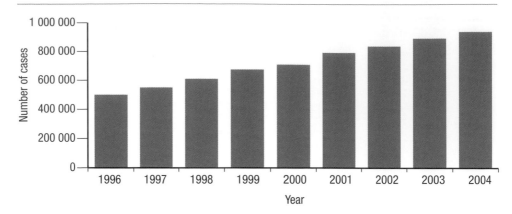

**FIGURE 9.6** Cases of chlamydia in the US 1996–2004.

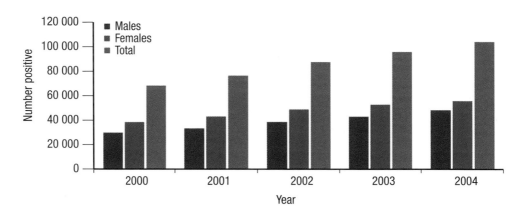

**FIGURE 9.7** Cases of genital chlamydia in the UK 2000–2004.

## Clinical history and examination

The incubation period is approximately one to three weeks. Around 50% of affected males are asymptomatic. Urethritis occurs in the other 50%.

## Diagnosis

*See* NGU. There are a number of DNA assays currently available for the diagnosis of chlamydia. These vary from country to country.

## Management

*See* NGU. It is important to note that chlamydia infection facilitates HIV transmission in men and women. There is increased detectable HIV virus in urethral secretions when infection is present. Partner notification is essential.

## KEY POINTS

▶ Most cases of penile discharge are due to sexually transmitted infection.
▶ Gonorrhoea and non-gonococcal urethritis remain a huge problem in both the developed and developing world.
▶ Partner notification is essential in all cases of sexually transmitted disease.

### CASE STUDY

Gary presented to the genito-urinary medicine clinic with a profuse, creamy penile discharge of three days duration. He denied sexual intercourse with anyone except his girlfriend. A gram stain of the pus obtained by a urethral swab demonstrated gram negative diplococci. Gary accepted treatment for gonorrhoea but refused to participate in partner notification and did not attend any follow up visits.

# 10

# HIV and AIDS

The management of patients with HIV and AIDS requires a specialised service. In the UK this is usually delivered by genito-urinary medicine physicians as part of a multi-disciplinary team. This chapter is not detailed but serves to raise awareness of this increasingly common infectious disease. If HIV or AIDS is suspected in a patient they should be referred for appropriate testing which requires pre-test counselling before investigations can be performed.

This chapter focuses on the male genitalia in HIV and AIDS and how infection with HIV may be suspected from genital skin disease and the presence of sexually transmitted infections.

The skin is one of the most important organs affected in patients with HIV. The number of skin disorders present in a patient with HIV is an indicator of the level of immunosuppression. Skin diseases in HIV cause considerable morbidity. Furthermore, the presence of skin disease is often the first clinical sign of HIV.

## Overview

The term 'acquired immunodeficiency syndrome' (AIDS) was coined in 1981 after cases of pneumocystis carinii (now called pneumocystis jiroveci) pneumonia were diagnosed in homosexual men in the US. The human immunodeficiency virus (HIV) responsible for infection was identified in 1983. There are two identified HIV viruses, HIV-1 and HIV-2. HIV-2 is predominantly found in West Africa. HIV is a lentivirus, a subgroup of the retrovirus family.

HIV targets CD4+ T lymphocytes and monocytes, resulting in reduced immune function. Progression from initial HIV infection to AIDS normally takes several years. The Centres for Disease Control and Prevention (CDC) produced a classification in 1993 for defining AIDS by a number of criteria.

| CD4+ T-cell categories | Clinical categories | | |
|---|---|---|---|
| | (A) Asymptomatic or PGL | (B) Symptomatic, not (A) or (C) conditions | (C) AIDS-indicator conditions |
| 1 ≥500/mm³ | A1 | B1 | C1 |
| 2 200–499/mm³ | A2 | B2 | C2 |
| 3 <200/mm³ | A3 | B3 | C3 |

NB Categories are defined by both CD4+ count and clinical presentation.
Shaded area indicates AIDS.
Where there is an overlap of conditions, (C) takes precedence over (B), which takes precedence over (A).
For classification purposes, once a category B condition has occurred, the subject will remain in category B. The same goes for progression to category C.

**Category A**
- Asymptomatic HIV infection
- Persistent generalised lymphadenopathy
- Acute (primary) HIV infection with accompanying illness or history of acute HIV infection

**Category B**
- Bacillary angiomatosis
- Candidiasis, oropharyngeal (thrush)
- Candidiasis, vulvovaginal; persistent, frequent or poorly responsive to therapy
- Cervical dysplasia (moderate or severe)/cervical carcinoma *in situ*
- Constitutional symptoms, such as fever (38.5°C) or diarrhoea lasting >1 month
- Hairy leucoplakia, oral
- Herpes zoster (shingles), involving at least two distinct episodes or more than one dermatome
- Idiopathic thrombocytopenic purpura
- Listeriosis
- Pelvic inflammatory disease, particularly if complicated by tuboovarian abscess
- Peripheral neuropathy

**Category C**
- Candidiasis of bronchi, trachea or lungs
- Candidiasis, oesophageal
- Cervical cancer, invasive
- Coccidioidomycosis, disseminated or extrapulmonary
- Cryptococcosis, extrapulmonary
- Cytomegalovirus disease (other than liver, spleen or nodes)
- Cytomegalovirus retinitis (with loss of vision)
- Encephalopathy, HIV-related
- Herpes simplex: chronic ulcer(s) (>1 month duration); or bronchitis, pneumonitis or oesophagitis
- Histoplasmosis, disseminated or extrapulmonary
- Isosporiasis, chronic intestinal (>1 month duration)
- Kaposi's sarcoma
- Lymphoma, Burkitt (or equivalent term)
- Lymphoma, primary, of brain
- *Mycobacterium avium* complex or *M. kansaii*, disseminated or extrapulmonary
- *Mycobacterium tuberculosis*, any site (pulmonary or extrapulmonary)
- *Mycobacterium*, other species or unidentified species, disseminated or extrapulmonary
- *Pneumocystis carinii* pneumonia
- Pneumonia, recurrent
- Progressive multifocal leucoencephalopathy
- *Salmonella* septicaemia, recurrent
- Toxoplasmosis of brain
- Wasting syndrome due to HIV

**FIGURE 10.1** Classification for defining AIDS (CDC 1993).

## Epidemiology

At the end of 2005, an estimated 40 million people worldwide were living with HIV infection. It is estimated there were around 14 000 new cases per day, mainly in developing countries. In (2006) there were around 62 000 people living with HIV in the UK, nearly half of them homosexual men. A quarter of all people with HIV in the UK are unaware of their infection. HIV was originally mainly confined to certain higher-risk groups, such as sex workers, homosexual men and intravenous drug addicts. However, in recent years this has changed with

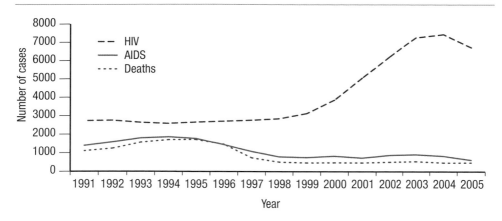

**FIGURE 10.2** Cases of HIV, AIDS and related deaths in the UK 1991–2005.

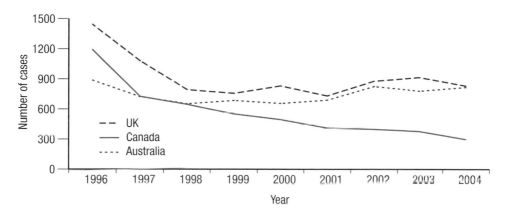

**FIGURE 10.3** HIV cases UK, Canada and Australia 1996–2004.

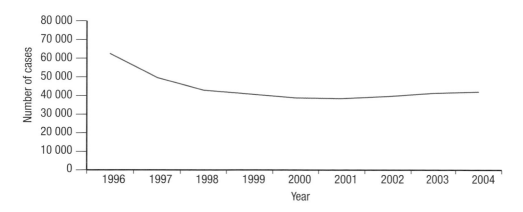

**FIGURE 10.4** New HIV cases United States 1996–2004.

more and more cases presenting in the heterosexual population. The number of heterosexuals newly diagnosed with HIV (58% of total) has increased since 1996. The number of new cases of HIV in the UK has doubled since 1998. Three quarters of heterosexual HIV infections diagnosed in the UK were acquired in Africa.

Some of the commonest skin manifestations associated with HIV and AIDS are listed below. Patients living with HIV tend to have a higher incidence of other sexually transmitted infections. These may present in much more unusual and florid forms than in patients without immunosuppression.

**TABLE 10.1** Genital skin problems and sexually transmitted infections commonly occurring in association with HIV

|  | Disease | See also |
| --- | --- | --- |
| **Skin manifestation** | Seborrhoeic dermatitis | Chapter 11, page 127 |
|  | Folliculitis | Chapter 2, page 21 |
|  | Psoriasis | Chapter 11, page 120 |
|  | Bacillary angiomatosis | Below |
|  | Sero-conversion illness | Below |
|  | Kaposi's sarcoma | Below |
| **Unusual presentation of sexually transmitted disease** | Molluscum contagiosum | Chapter 5, page 52 |
|  | Syphilis | Chapter 8, page 83 |
|  | Genital warts | Chapter 5, page 49 |
|  | Herpes simplex virus | Chapter 8, page 90 |
|  | Scabies | Chapter 3, page 28 |

## COMMON SKIN MANIFESTATIONS OF HIV AND AIDS THAT MAY PRESENT IN THE GENITAL AREA

### Seborrhoeic eczema

Seborrhoeic eczema is usually the first skin manifestation of HIV infection, tending to affect the naso-labial folds most commonly. The extent of the eruption may be more widespread than in non-HIV individuals. In longstanding HIV infection where immune function is severely compromised, seborrhoeic eczema may be extremely severe at the classical sites such as the face or may present as a generalised rash when the differential diagnosis will include widespread eczema, psoriasis or dermatophytosis.

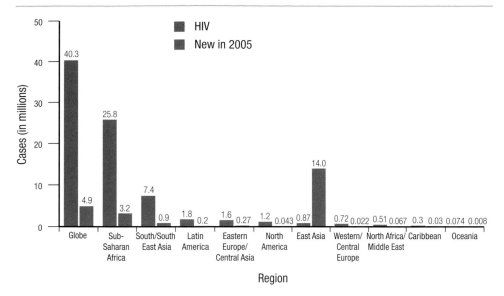

**FIGURE 10.5** HIV: a world perspective.

## Folliculitis

Due to reduced immune function, folliculitis tends to be more common in HIV patients. Bacterial folliculitis, particularly caused by staphylococcus aureus is a problem in the groins in men.

There is a rare form of folliculitis almost exclusive to men with HIV called eosinophilic folliculitis. It tends to occur relatively early in HIV infection when CD4+ counts are around $250–300 \times 10^6$/L. Classically, patients have an itchy rash with recurrent crops of sterile pustules centred on hair follicles, mainly on the face and trunk. Phototherapy has been used successfully.

## Psoriasis

Patients with HIV with pre-existing psoriasis may develop a significant flare of their skin. Psoriasis may also present for the first time in HIV. It tends to be severe and more difficult to manage than in patients without immunosuppression. In addition, the morphology may be atypical. Psoriasis may actually regress in the pre-terminal stages of HIV infection, although the mechanism for this is unclear. Genital psoriasis may be the only manifestation of the disease in HIV. Since psoriasis tends to be worse when the skin is irritated or traumatised (the Koebner phenomenon) severe skin problems in the genital area such as intertrigo or herpes infection may precipitate or exacerbate the disease.

Caution with topical steroids in the genital area is necessary in HIV patients due to the risk of reactivation or worsening of pre-existing infections. Most patients do well with conventional psoriasis therapies although immunosuppressive agents such as ciclosporin and methotrexate should be avoided.

### Bacillary angiomatosis

This rare skin condition has important associations with HIV. The disease is caused by Bartonella species, a gram negative bacillus. One study of AIDS patients revealed subjects ranging from 26 to 52 years were infected. Patients often have symptoms for many months before a diagnosis is made. Constitutional symptoms such as fever, weight loss and anorexia may occur. Lesions present as papules and nodules. They may be small multiple red lesions resembling pyogenic granulomas or may be larger, solitary and resemble Kaposi's sarcoma. Diagnosis may be rapidly made using PCR enzyme immunoassay.

### Sero-conversion illness

Sero-conversion illnesses tend to have similar symptoms and the majority of cases of primary HIV infection will not come to the attention of the medical profession. Symptoms tend to be non-specific and include sore throat, fever and lymph node enlargement. Tiredness, arthralgia and myalgia are common as is a non-itchy polymorphic erythematous rash (found in up to three quarters of patients with symptomatic sero-conversion). The illness may be confused with Epstein Barr infection (infectious mononucleosis) as well as a range of other infectious and inflammatory diseases. Non-specific genital ulceration may be a presentation of primary HIV infection.

### Kaposi's sarcoma

This rare skin tumour is an AIDS-defining condition and is the most common neoplastic disease in AIDS patients. Prior to the 1980s, Kaposi's sarcoma (KS) was classified into three groups: 'classic' KS found mainly in elderly Jewish or Eastern European men, 'endemic' or African KS and immunosuppression-related KS found in transplant patients. The disease is caused by the human herpes virus type 8 (also known as Kaposi's sarcoma-associated herpes virus).

The penis is a common skin site for lesions, as is the head and neck and the soles of the feet. Lesions tend to vary in size up to several centimetres in diameter and are usually multiple. They vary in colour from red-brown to blue. Kaposi's sarcoma can not be cured due to the disseminated nature of lesions. Both chemotherapy and radiotherapy have been used for palliation.

# COMMON ASSOCIATED SEXUALLY TRANSMITTED INFECTIONS
## Molluscum contagiosum

Widespread molluscum contagiosum, particularly giant lesions, are usually considered a marker for HIV infection. As with other skin conditions in HIV, the clinical presentation may be variable and diagnosis may be difficult. The classical umbilicated papules seen normally may not be evident. Molluscum may be confused with basal cell carcinoma, keratoacanthoma and some skin infections. Where there is any debate about diagnosis a skin biopsy for histological analysis should be taken. Lesions may be extremely resistant to therapy, although treatment with HAART is often helpful. Molluscum in adults on the face and chest should raise the possibility of HIV infection.

## Syphilis

The presence of syphilitic chancres makes it easier to transmit and acquire HIV sexually. The risk of acquiring HIV is estimated to be increased two- to fivefold when syphilis is present. It is common for the two diseases to co-exist and co-infected patients show slower resolution of primary chancres. The

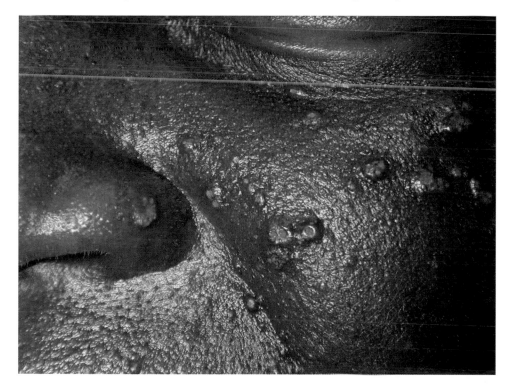

**FIGURE 10.6** Molluscum on the face of a patient with HIV.

reduced immune function of HIV patients means that eradication of syphilis may be difficult in some cases, particularly if there is central nervous system involvement.

The features of secondary syphilis may be more pronounced in HIV patients. However, the existence of rashes known to be associated with HIV such as drug rashes, eosinophilic folliculitis, oral lesions and oral ulceration and condylomata, may make the clinical diagnosis of secondary syphilis difficult.

## Genital warts

Patients with HIV are more prone to developing clinically-evident lesions of genital warts. In addition, they may suffer complications such as the development of giant condylomata or pre-malignant lesions. Extensive warts may be an indicator of HIV.

## Herpes simplex

If the HIV patient's immune system is relatively intact the clinical presentation of

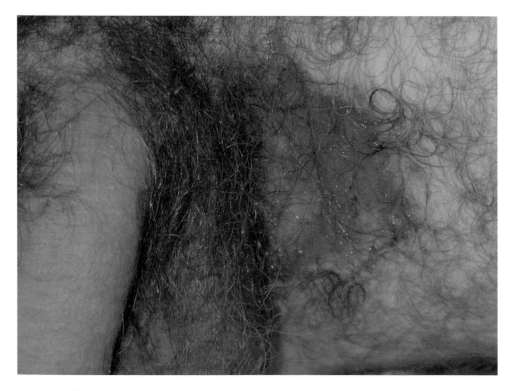

**FIGURE 10.7** Severe localised herpes simplex of the groin in a man with HIV infection.

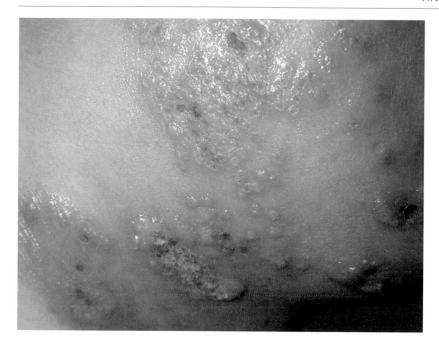

**FIGURE 10.8** Severe and extensive herpes simplex infection of the face.

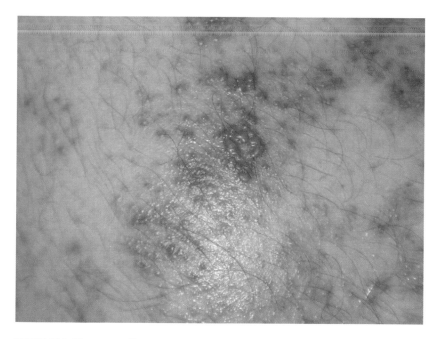

**FIGURE 10.9** Close up of herpes simplex vesicles.

herpes simplex will be the same as in patients with a normal immune function. Herpes simplex should be a differential diagnosis in ulceration of any type in HIV patients.

Herpes simplex infection in HIV tends to be more frequently recurrent and more severe. Lesions may become chronic with persistent painful ulceration of the skin. Management has become easier since the advent of highly active antiretroviral treatment (HAART). Aciclovir resistance is an increasing problem in patients with HIV and AIDS, usually due to thymidine kinase-negative aciclovir-resistant HSV type 2.

Herpes simplex may cause a necrotising folliculitis of the skin. This presents as small crusty non-healing papules.

## Scabies

Although classical scabies is common in HIV patients, crusted or Norwegian scabies is also a major problem. The condition is highly contagious. The patient is infected with millions of mites and is likely to be resistant to topical therapy alone. Ivermectin at 200 microgram/kg as a single oral dose is effective. It should be noted that both scabies and pubic lice can not pass on the HIV virus from one patient to another.

Scabies in HIV patients may be confused with other inflammatory scaling conditions such as seborrhoeic eczema and psoriasis. There may be evidence of lesions on the head and neck.

## KEY POINTS

) HIV is increasing rapidly across many countries of the world.
) Skin lesions may be the first sign of HIV.
) HIV should be considered a possibility in all patients with sexually transmitted diseases, especially where the presentation is unusual.

**CASE STUDY**

Max, a heterosexual, married 52-year-old man, attended the dermatology clinic with a six month history of florid eczema. He admitted to 2 stones in weight loss over this period. He had a widespread eczema but also severe oral candidosis. A full blood count revealed a pancytopenia. Although he appeared to have no risk factors for HIV infection, he was offered screening after appropriate counselling. The HIV test was positive and his CD4$^+$ cell count was only 54. He was started on HAART which resulted in a rapid improvement in his skin disease and a rise in his CD4$^+$ count. He remains under regular follow up under the care of his local genito-urinary medicine clinic.

# 11

# Common skin conditions affecting the genitals

Many skin conditions affect the genitals. It is not uncommon for patients to be too embarrassed to bring this to the attention of their doctor. Unfortunately, even in dermatology clinics the genitals may not be examined when a patient presents with a widespread skin eruption. There are a number of common skin conditions that often have a genital component which may be quite different to the appearance of the disease elsewhere on the body. The two most common skin problems with potential genital involvement are eczema and psoriasis. The following skin diseases commonly present on the genitals:

- psoriasis
- eczema: contact irritant, allergic contact and seborrhoeic forms
- acanthosis nigricans
- lichen sclerosus (*see* Chapter 4, page 38)
- Reiter's syndrome (*see* Chapter 6, page 73)
- lichen planus (*see* Chapter 6, page 69).

One of the problems of genital dermatoses in men is that their appearance can be non-specific, especially in non-circumcised individuals. This may cause confusion in diagnosis. Chronic, unremitting dermatoses of the genitals, particularly those not responding to appropriate therapy may be the presentation of a malignant or pre-malignant condition such as Bowen's disease or extra-mammary Paget's disease (*see* Chapter 2, page 19).

## PSORIASIS

Psoriasis is a common, chronic eruption, characterised by symmetrical, scaly plaques. Although the skin is the primary organ affected, around 10% of patients also have some joint involvement. The disease often first presents in teenage years. There is a strong genetic component to psoriasis.

### Incidence

At least 2% of the UK and US population are affected. In the US it is estimated there are around 200 000–250 000 new cases per year. The disease is less common in the tropics.

### Clinical history and examination

Psoriasis of the genitals may present with soreness, irritation and itching, particularly of the groins and the glans penis. Patients may be alarmed by the appearance of a red penile rash.

Psoriasis on the genitals may be the only presentation of the disease on the skin. However, careful examination of patients usually reveals skin lesions elsewhere. Psoriasis presents as erythematous plaques with a silvery scale. Lesions vary from just a few millimetres in diameter to many centimetres. The eruption tends to be symmetrical, particularly on the extensor surfaces of the body. Nail changes are common with features such as pitting, onycholysis and subungual hyperkeratosis. Genital psoriasis tends not to be itchy, but may be sore.

It is relatively common for psoriasis to affect the flexures (natal cleft, groins), perianal skin and the shaft, glans and prepuce of the penis. In the circumcised man the lesions tend to be typical plaques (*see* Figures 11.1 and 11.4). In the uncircumcised man the appearance may resemble a non-specific balanitis with only mild or no scaling present.

It is important to recognise that psoriasis may be extremely severe in patients with HIV. Falling immune function may reveal and worsen psoriasis in these patients.

### Diagnosis

The diagnosis is usually made clinically. In the uncircumcised man diagnosis can be difficult and skin biopsy may be helpful. In such patients the differential diagnosis may include Zoon's balanitis, extra-mammary Paget's disease and lichen planus.

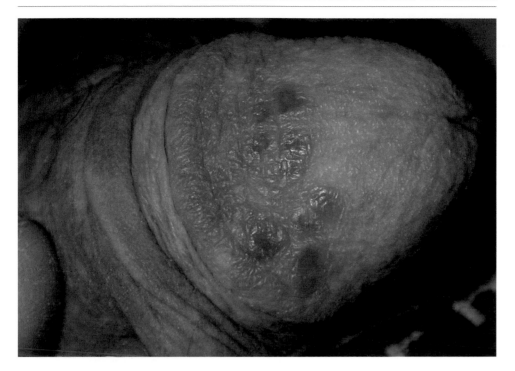

FIGURE 11.1 Small plaques of psoriasis on the glans penis (lesions may resemble lichen planus).

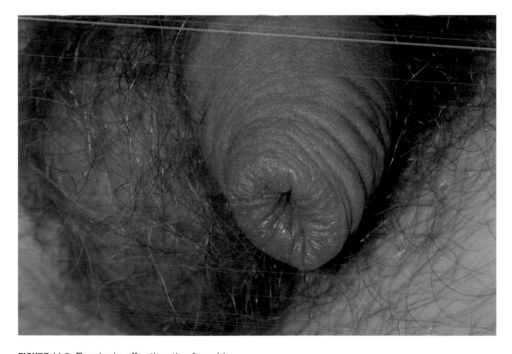

FIGURE 11.2 Psoriasis affecting the foreskin.

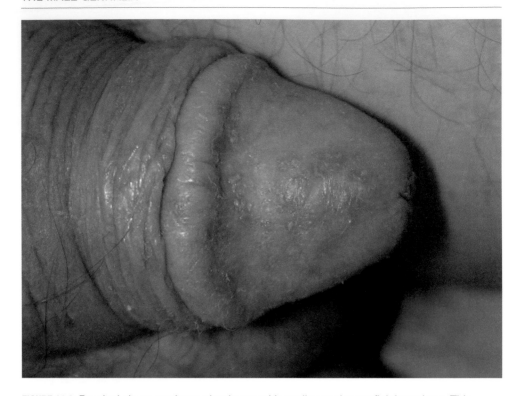

**FIGURE 11.3** Psoriasis in an uncircumcised man with scaling and superficial erosions. This appearance is very similar to the balanitis seen in Reiter's syndrome.

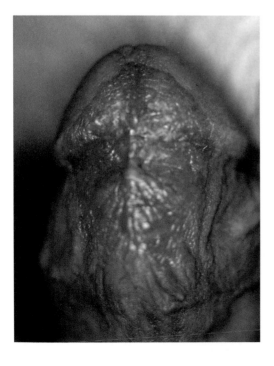

**FIGURE 11.4** Localised plaque of psoriasis.

## Management

Men with genital psoriasis are often extremely embarrassed about their condition and may fail to mention their symptoms to medical staff. Reassurance is important. Standard treatment involves the use of topical emollients, soap substitutes and topical steroids for limited periods. Unfortunately, most topical therapies designed for psoriasis are too irritant for the genital skin. It is unusual for systemic therapies to be needed for genital psoriasis alone.

## ECZEMA

Eczema on the genitals may be classified as exogenous (allergic contact dermatitis or irritant contact dermatitis) or endogenous (atopic eczema or seborrhoeic eczema). Other forms of eczema on the genitals are exceptionally rare.

## Allergic contact dermatitis

As the name suggests, this form of eczema is caused by direct contact with a sensitising substance. The reaction is in the form of a type IV (delayed type) hypersensitivity. Allergens may be applied directly to the skin (for example in the form of a cream), or may be transferred from elsewhere (for example by the hands after handling an allergic substance).

Symptoms may be acute, chronic or acute-on-chronic. Acute contact dermatitis of the genital skin usually presents with redness, itching and swelling. In severe cases the skin may blister and there may be exudation. This reaction tends to occur within 24 to 48 hours after contact with a sensitising agent. With intermittent exposure to an offending allergen a chronic, irritating, lichenified eczema may develop (see lichenified eczema below).

Investigation with patch testing is essential. Treatment involves withdrawing offending allergens if known, avoiding irritants (such as soap) and the use of moderately potent topical steroids for limited periods.

Type IV reactions to latex may occur but are relatively rare. Most reactions to rubber are due to allergy to the rubber chemicals (e.g. accelerators). Type I reactions to rubber in the form of latex reactions are important since they may be very severe or even life threatening. These reactions may cause acute (within minutes) urticaria, swelling, irritation and redness of the skin but may also precipitate acute anaphylaxis.

**TABLE 11.1** Common sources of allergic contact dermatitis on the genitalia

| Where allergen originates from | Source | Examples | Specific sensitisers |
|---|---|---|---|
| **Direct contact** | Medicaments and skin care products | Topical steroids, emollients, local anaesthetic creams, antibiotics, antifungals, bath products | Parabens, ethylene diamine, sorbic acid, propylene glycol etc. |
| | Contraceptives | Condoms | Latex, spermicides, rubber chemicals |
| **Allergen transfer** | Hands | Industrial allergens | Nickel, epoxies |
| | Partner | Feminine products | Fragrances |

## Irritant contact dermatitis

Irritant contact dermatitis may be clinically indistinguishable from allergic contact dermatitis. There are a large number of potential irritants (*see* below), particularly soaps, shower gels and bath products which are often highly fragranced. Poor hygiene is often a predisposing factor, especially in older men.

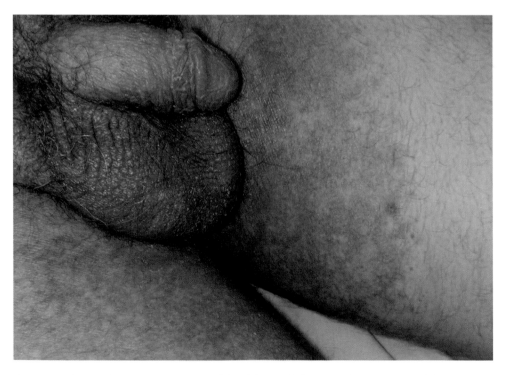

**FIGURE 11.5** Acute allergic contact dermatitis of the genital area and surrounding skin. Note the sharp demarcation of the rash.

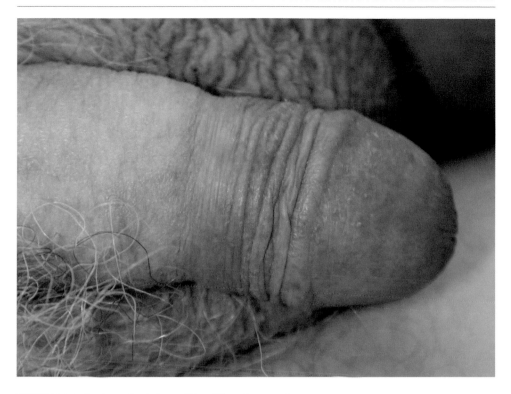

**FIGURE 11.6** Irritant contact dermatitis of the glans and prepuce.

Typical irritants of the genital area:
- soaps, shower gels and other toiletries
- urine, faeces
- sweat, sebum
- condoms, spermicides, products to enhance sex
- sexual secretions
- tight clothing and friction.

Management of irritant contact dermatitis is similar to that of allergic contact dermatitis with avoidance of all irritant factors, use of appropriate emollients and soap substitutes and limited use of a topical steroid.

## Atopic eczema and lichen simplex

Atopic eczema (atopic dermatitis) is very common, affecting around 10% of children, although only a small percentage will continue to have problems into adulthood. In moderate and severe cases the eruption may be widespread and

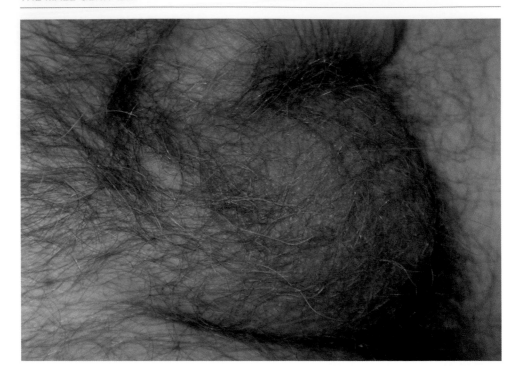

**FIGURE 11.7** Scrotal eczema with erythema and mild scaling (clinically this could be irritant dermatitis or seborrhoeic dermatitis).

affect the genital area. It is unusual for atopic eczema to be only confined to the genitals and lesions will invariably be visible elsewhere on the body. This group of patients are more prone to contact allergy (*see* above) and patch testing may be useful in their management. Treatment is the same for allergic contact dermatitis and irritant contact dermatitis.

Lichen simplex is the term given to describe chronic, lichenified eczema of any variety. It is very common in the groins and on the scrotum where it is produced by scratching and rubbing. It may develop into intertrigo (*see* Chapter 2) and may be complicated by bacterial or fungal infection, particularly in the groins. General advice such as keeping the fingernails short is important. Treatment is similar to that of the other forms of eczema but due to the intense itch, potent topical steroids may be necessary for a longer period. Secondary infection should be treated concurrently.

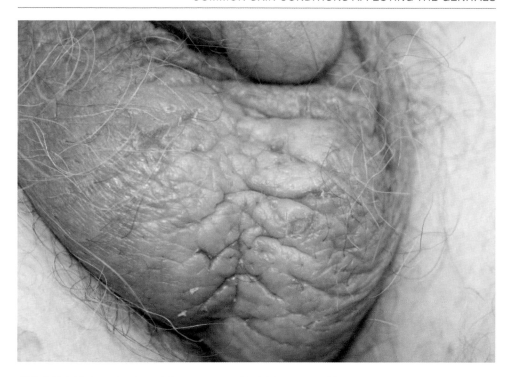

**FIGURE 11.8** Lichen simplex of the scrotum with thickening and fissuring of the scrotal skin.

## Seborrhoeic eczema (Seborrhoeic dermatitis)

Seborrhoeic eczema is a papulosquamous skin disorder usually localised to specific sebum-rich areas of the body such as the face, scalp and trunk, but also occurs in hairy areas such as the pubic area. It occurs worldwide and at a higher rate in men than women. The prevalence is estimated at around 5% in healthy individuals but occurs in up to 85% of HIV-infected patients. It is associated with an abnormal immune response to the Malassezia yeast species.

Symptoms may be mild or absent. Mild itching, tingling or even burning of the skin may occur. Erythema, scaling and crusting are present to variable degrees. The eruption may be confined to the genital area but closer examination will often reveal signs elsewhere, such as dandruff in the scalp and mild scaling affecting the naso-labial folds, eyebrows and eyelash areas.

Seborrhoeic eczema is usually the first cutaneous manifestation of HIV infection. In longstanding HIV infection where immune function is severely compromised, seborrhoeic eczema may be very severe or generalised.

Diagnosis is usually made clinically but skin scrapings may be necessary to exclude tinea. The yeast will be visible on microscopy. The differential diagnosis includes genital psoriasis (which may also co-exist), other forms of eczema and fungal infections. Standard therapies tend to combine a mild topical steroid with an antifungal agent, as well as the use of emollients and soap substitutes. Unfortunately, the yeast can not be completely eradicated and the eruption tends to recur periodically.

## ACANTHOSIS NIGRICANS

This is a common disorder characterised by a velvety thickening and pigmentation of the skin. It is usually localised to the axillae, groins and nape of the neck. It is most commonly associated with obesity and is more common in people with dark skins. It may be an incidental finding affecting the groins when examining the genitalia in men. Although most cases are related to obesity and insulin resistance, there are cases related to internal malignancy and other factors such as drugs.

## KEY POINTS

❱ Many common skin conditions may affect the genitalia.
❱ Rashes on the glans penis are often non-specific in uncircumcised men.
❱ It is important to ask about a personal and family history of skin disease in men with genital problems.
❱ Examination of the rest of the skin will often facilitate diagnosis.

---

**CASE STUDY**

A 29-year-old Asian man attended a diabetic clinic. It was noted he was grossly overweight. He complained of numerous skin tags around his axillae and a discolouration of the skin in his groins. Examination revealed the typical changes of acanthosis nigricans in the groins and axillae with dark, velvety thickened skin in both regions. Unfortunately, despite good diabetic control and weight loss there was no improvement in the appearance of his skin after several months.

# 12

# Psychological and psychiatric disorders

Patients with significant psychological and psychiatric problems may present with genital symptoms. The general practitioner, genito-urinary physician and dermatologist must be aware of this small percentage of patients who are exceedingly difficult to treat. When disease or perceived disease affects the genital area, the psychological aspects may be overwhelming. Healthcare staff may feel unable to deal with such patients, particularly in the absence of disease and a referral to psychological or psychiatric services may be necessary. This is very important if depression or a suicide risk is a possibility. Some specialist clinics run a joint dermatology and psychological or psychiatric service.

There are a number of psychological and psychiatric conditions that may present with genital symptoms:

- dysaesthesia syndromes, e.g. burning scrotal syndrome, burning penis syndrome, red scrotum syndrome
- dermatitis artefacta (self-inflicted injury)
- dysmorphophobia (altered body perception)
- delusions of parasitosis.

## DYSAESTHESIA SYNDROMES

So-called 'dysaesthesia' syndromes include a range of conditions where the predominant symptom is altered skin sensation, particularly burning and pain. This may involve the penis, scrotum or both. There is usually no sign of skin disease. The condition in men is rarely reported in the literature unlike the synonymous condition of vulvodynia in women. There is an association with child sexual abuse in some patients. There are case reports suggesting zinc deficiency (in acrodermatitis enteropathica) may be a differential diagnosis. Reassurance is usually unhelpful but there is evidence that antidepressants may be of some benefit. As with all psychological and psychiatric problems referral to a relevant specialist may help significantly.

## DERMATITIS ARTEFACTA (SELF-INFLICTED SKIN DISEASE)

Dermatitis artefacta occurs two to three times more commonly in females compared with males. Self-harm directed at the genital area is rare. Inconsistencies in the clinical history may alert the clinician to the possibility of the condition. Skin lesions commonly appear within hours. The patient may be emotionally immature or may have an obvious psychological problem. It is not uncommon for such patients to have a degree of medical knowledge.

Lesions of dermatitis artefacta usually do not conform to known dermatoses. They may be linear, angular or in a geometric pattern. They are usually inflammatory and may present as red areas, blisters, ulcers or erosions. Patients may use a variety of instruments to harm themselves including lit cigarettes, knives, pins, hot items and so forth.

Management is extremely difficult. The lesions must first be treated medically by antibiotics, topical agents, dressings and so on. However, early specialist psychological intervention is important. Many of these patients are considered to have a suicide risk. Direct confrontation is not recommended since the patients will usually deny self-harm. Unfortunately, patients often refuse any psychiatric or psychological therapy.

## DYSMORPHOPHOBIA (BODY DYSMORPHIC SYNDROME)

Dysmorphophobia is an uncommon but difficult-to-treat condition. The imagined defects in appearance are often focused on the genitals. The ICD-10 definition is:

1. Persistent belief in the presence of at least one serious physical illness underlying the presenting symptom(s), even though repeated investigations and examinations have identified no adequate physical explanation, or a persistent preoccupation with a presumed deformity or disfigurement.
2. Persistent refusal to accept the advice and reassurance of several different doctors that there is no physical illness or abnormality underlying the symptoms.

Most studies have shown more men than women are affected. There is recent evidence suggesting an increase in the number of men suffering from dysmorphophobia associated with so-called 'life-style' drug use such as finasteride. Some studies suggest the rate of dysmorphophobia is relatively high in patients seeking dermatological treatment.

The symptoms of body dysmorphic syndrome can vary. Perception of body asymmetry is common. Attention may be focused on normal anatomical variants of the genitalia. Patients tend to have low self-esteem, feelings of embarrassment, shame and fear of rejection. Insight is usually absent. The following questions may aid diagnosis:

- Have you ever been worried about your appearance? What was your concern?
- Did this worry or pre-occupy you? Did you think a lot about it and wish you could worry about it less?
- What effect on your life has this had? Has it caused you much distress or has it affected your work, social life family, friends or any other activities?

The condition is extremely difficult to manage. Repeated reassurance and investigation is unhelpful. Social impairment is common, stress levels are high and quality of life in affected individuals is significantly reduced. Associated major depression, suicidal ideation and obsessive-compulsive disorder are very common. Most authorities agree the best current therapy is with a combination of psychotherapy and psychopharmacological treatment. Unfortunately, of the little follow up research that has been performed, data suggests a relatively poor prognosis.

## DELUSIONS OF PARASITOSIS

In this condition the patient has the firm belief that they are infested with insects or other parasites. Patients may present in the dermatology clinic with widespread itching or very rarely with a delusional belief that genital symptoms are related to infestation. The term is used to describe those patients who appear to have a fixed hypochondriacal delusion that is not related to any other psychiatric illness. However, delusions of parasitosis may occasionally be a secondary feature of other psychiatric illnesses such as schizophrenia, depression and anxiety disorders.

When delusions of parasitosis are focused on the genitals there may be a history of unprotected sexual intercourse with an individual other than the patient's regular partner. As with the other psychological and psychiatric conditions that may present with a skin complaint, patients are often unwilling to accept medical advice and reassurance and will seek several opinions. Symptoms of itching, burning and 'crawling under the skin' are common. There may be excoriations, scars or gouges in the skin where the patient has attempted to remove the imaginary parasites. The patient may also have subjected himself to extreme cleansing routines with insecticides, disinfectants and other harsh substances. Otherwise, the skin will be normal on examination. It is common also for the patient to bring 'evidence' of their infestation in the form of crusts, dust and fragments of hair, clothing and other substances.

As with the other conditions in this chapter, it is important to keep an open mind to the possibility of organic disease (e.g. scabies). Some investigation may be required to exclude organic illnesses. Pimozide was the treatment of choice for this condition in the past but newer medications such as risperidone are now in use. Psychiatric supervision is usually necessary if the patient will accept referral.

## KEY POINTS

❭ Consider a psychological problem in patients with severe symptoms but no evidence of organic disease.
❭ Psychological and psychiatric disease presenting with genital symptoms is extremely difficult to treat and the intervention of a psychiatrist or psychologist is often necessary.
❭ Patients with these problems are often vulnerable. Tact and understanding is needed when treating them.

### CASE STUDY

Roland, a 45-year-old salesman, had persistent burning of his penis for three months. He was convinced he had something seriously wrong with him despite the assurance of three trips to the local genito-urinary department.

He was referred to the dermatology clinic by his general practitioner. No abnormalities of the skin were found. Roland was a nervous man, fastidious and well turned out. He remained convinced there was something wrong despite further reassurances.

On Roland's second visit to the dermatology clinic he offered the information that he thought he may have a sexually transmitted disease after having had a one-night stand with a woman on one of his business trips. When it was pointed out that the time of onset of his penile symptoms was just a day following this sexual encounter Roland realised the symptoms were psychosomatic. Within four weeks he was symptom-free, although he continued to get occasional flare-ups for some time.

# Appendices

## APPENDIX 1: COMMON DERMATOLOGICAL TERMS

| | |
|---|---|
| Abscess | a collection of pus |
| Atrophy | loss of epidermis and/or dermis |
| Bulla | a fluid-filled blister over 5mm diameter |
| Crust | dried exudate on the skin surface |
| Cyst | a skin nodule made up of an epithelial-lined cavity filled with a fluid or more solid material |
| Erosion | a superficial loss of epidermis that heals without scarring |
| Erythema | skin redness |
| Excoriation | epidermal damage due to scratching |
| Filiform | finger-like projections from the skin |
| Hyperkeratotic | thickening (hypertrophy) of the stratum corneum |
| Hypertrophy | an increase in the size of a cell or organ (in the skin it relates to epidermal and/or dermal increase) |
| Keloid | a raised scar |
| Lichenification | thickening of the skin with attenuated skin markings |
| Macule | a flat area of colour change |
| Nodule | a large papule, typically more than 1cm diameter |
| Papule | a raised lesion, typically less than 1cm diameter |
| Plaque | a circumscribed raised area, typically more than 2cm diameter |
| Pustule | a pus-filled blister |
| Scale | an accumulation of keratin on the skin surface |
| Vesicle | a fluid-filled blister less than 5mm diameter |
| Wheal (weal) | a raised area of skin caused by dermal oedema |

| Ulcer | a loss of cells extending through the epidermis and into the dermis. |

## APPENDIX 2: USEFUL WEBSITES AND PATIENT SUPPORT GROUPS

**UK**

**Acne Support Group**
Howard House
The Runway
South Ruislip
Middlesex HA4 6SE
Tel: 0870 870 2263
Website: www.stopspots.org

**Behcet's Syndrome Society**
3 Church Close
Lambourn
Hingerford
Berks RG17 8PU
Tel: 01488 71116
Website: www.behcets.org.uk
Email: info@behcets-society.fsnet.co.uk

**Darier's Disease Support Group**
29 St Annes Road
Hakin
Milford Haven
Pembrokeshire SA73 3LQ
Tel: 01646 695055
Website: www.dariers.com

**Everyman (Male cancers)**
The Institute of Cancer Research
Freepost LON 922
London SW7 3YY
Tel: 0800 731 9468
Website: http://www.icr.ac.uk/everyman/
Email: everyman@icr.ac.uk

**Hairline International – The Alopecia Patient's Society**
Lyons Court
1668 High Street
Knowle
West Midlands B93 0LY
Tel: 01564 775281
Website: www.hairlineinternational.co.uk

**The Herpes Viruses Association**
41 North Road
London N7 9DP
Tel: 020 7609 9061
Website: www.herpes.org.uk
Email: info@herpes.org.uk

**Men's Health Forum**
Tavistock House
Tavistock Square
London WC1H 9HR
Tel: 020 7388 4449
Website: www.menshealthforum.org.uk

**Men's Health Line**
Medical Advisory Service
PO Box 3087
London W4 4ZP
Tel: 020 8995 4448
Website: http://www.hkmenshealth.com/eng/healthline/index.asp

**National AIDS Helpline**
1st Floor
Cavern Court
8 Matthews Street
Liverpool L2 6RE
Tel: 0151 227 4150

**National AIDS Trust**
196 Old Street
London EC1V 9FR
Tel: 020 7814 6767
Website: www.nat.org.uk

**National Eczema Society**
Hill House
Highgate Hill
London N19 5NA
Tel: 0870 241 3604
Website: www.eczema.org
Email: eczemapro@eczema.org

**National Lichen Sclerosus Support Group**
PO Box 5830
Lyme Regis
Dorset DT7 3ZU
Website: www.lichensclerosus.org

**The Psoriasis Association**
7 Milton Street
Northampton NN2 7JG
Tel: 01604 711129
Website: www.psoriasis-association.org.uk
Email: mail@psoriasis.demon.co.uk

**Shingles Support Society**
41 North Road
London N7 9DP
Website: www.herpes.org.uk

**The Terrence Higgins Trust (HIV & AIDS)**
52–54 Gray's Inn Road
London WC1X 8JU
Tel: 020 7242 1010
Website: www.tht.org.uk
Email: into@tht.org.uk

**The Vitiligo Society**
125 Kennington Road
London SE11 6SF
Tel: 0800 0182631
Website: www.vitiligosociety.org.uk
Email: all@vitiligosociety.org.uk

## European

### International Society for Men's Health

PO Box 46
A-1097 Vienna
Tel: +43 1 409 60 10-0
Website: www.ismh.org
Email: office@ismh.org

## US & Canada

### American Skin Association

150 East 58th Street
33rd Floor
New York MY 10155-0002
Tel: (212) 753 8260

### American Social Health Association (ASHA)

PO Box 13827
Research Triangle Park
NC 27709-3827
Tel: 1 800 783 9877
Website: www.ashastd.org

### Canadian Psoriasis Foundation

1565 Carling Avenue
1306 Wellington Street
Suite 500F
Ottawa, Ontario
Canada K1Y 3B2
Tel: (613) 728 4000

### Division of STD prevention (DSTDP)

Centres for Disease Control and Prevention
Website: www.cdc.gov/std

### Herpes Resource Centre

American Social Health Association
PO Box 13827
Research Triangle Park
NC 27709
Tel: (919) 361 8488
Website: http://sunsite.unc.edu/ASHA/

## Men's Health Network

PO Box 75972
Washington DC 20013
Tel: (202) 543 6461
Website: www.menshealthnetwork.org
Email: info@menshealthnetwork.org

## National Alopecia Areata Foundation

6600 SW 92nd Avenue
Suite 300
Portland OR 97223-7195
Tel: (503) 244 7404
Website: www.psoriasis.org

## National Eczema Association for Science & Education

1220 SW Morrison Street
Suite 433
Portland OR 97205
Tel: (503) 228 4430
Website: www.eczema-assn.org

## National Herpes Resource Center

Website: http://www.ashastd.org/herpes/herpes_overview.cfm
Email: herpesnet@ashastd.org

## National Pediculosis Association

PO Box 149
Newton MA 02161
Tel: (617) 449 6487
Website: www.headlice.org

## National Psoriasis Foundation

6600 SW 92nd Avenue
Suite 300
Portland OR 97223-7195
Tel: (503) 244 7404
Website: www.psoriasis.org/npf.shtml

## National Vitiligo Foundation

PO Box 6117
Tyler TX 75711
Tel: (903) 595 3713

Website: www.nvfi.org
Email: info@nvfi.org

**Psoriasis Society of Canada**
National Office
PO Box 25015
Halifax
Canada NS B3M 4H4
Tel: 902 443 8680

**STD information and referrals to STD Clinics**
CDC-INFO
Tel: 1-800-CDC-INFO (800 232 4636)

**VZV Research Foundation (Shingles & Post-herpetic neuralgia)**
36 East 72nd Street
New York NY 10021
Tel: (212) 472 3181

## Professional societies

**American Academy of Dermatology**
930 North Meacham Road
PO Box 4014
Schaumburg IL 60168-4014
Tel: (847) 330 0230
Website: www.aad.org

**American Dermatology Foundation**
1560 Sherman Avenue
Suite 302
Evanston IL 60201-4802
Tel: 708 328 2256

**American Society for Dermatological Surgery**
5550 Meadowbrook Drive
Suite 120
Rolling Meadows IL 60008
Tel: (847) 956 0900
Website: www.asds-net.org
Email:  info@asds.net

**British Association of Dermatologists**
19 Fitzroy Square
London W1P 5HQ
Tel: 020 7383 0266
Website: www.bad.org

**European Academy of Dermatology & Venereology**
38 Avenue General de Gaulle
B-1050 Brussels
Belgium
Tel: 32 265 00 90
Website: www.eadv.org
Email: office@eadv.org

**International Foundation for Dermatology**
855 West 10th
Vancouver BC V5Z 1L7
Canada
Tel: (604) 874 6112

**International Union against Sexually Transmitted Infections**
Website: www.iusti.org

**New Zealand Dermatological Society**
2 Fairdene Avenue
Henderson
Auckland
Tel: 09 524 5011
Website: www.dermnetnz.org

## APPENDIX 3:   'PARTNER NOTIFICATION' (CONTACT TRACING)

Partner notification is an important aspect of the management of sexually transmitted diseases and should be carried out by personnel trained in various aspects of sexual health. The same skills needed to take a full sexual history (*see* Chapter 1, page 4) are needed for partner notification, as is knowledge and experience of the local community, communication skills and knowledge of legal and social issues.

The aims of partner notification are:
- to ensure that contacts of patients with sexually transmitted infections are informed so that they can receive testing, counselling and treatment

- to reduce the risk of re-infection as far as the index patient is concerned
- to reduce the prevalence of infection in the community
- enable early testing and treatment before complications develop.

Some sexually transmitted diseases such as hepatitis B, gonorrhoea and early stage syphilis are highly contagious and in such cases contact tracing is a high priority. The infected patient is asked to give his or her sexual partners a note (contact slip) asking them to come to the sexual health clinic. The note will usually contain details of the patient's case number, clinical diagnosis (in code form) and the date of diagnosis. All patients with sexually transmitted infections that could lead to significant morbidity in an untreated sexual partner should be counselled with a view to participate in partner notification.

Important infections that require partner notification include:
- Chlamydia
- Gonorrhoea
- Syphilis
- Epididymitis in sexually active young men (<35 years)
- Non specific urethritis
- Hepatitis B and C
- HIV.

## APPENDIX 4:   CONFIDENTIAL COUNSELLING

Important aspects to consider in order to achieve successful counselling via an index patient would include giving information the following:
- the condition(s)
- possibilities of reinfection
- treatment proposed and efficacy
- possible complications if untreated
- safer sex advice (including the use of barrier methods and the duration of sexual abstinence)
- advice on the silent nature of most sexually transmitted diseases
- indicate the long term damage of delay in treatment from the partner's point of view as well as a public health point of view.

In addition, reassurance should be given that all information would be treated with strict confidentiality. If the index patient is not willing to undertake to inform the partner/s, the need to resort to the health care provider (Health advisor) to do the contacting should be highlighted.

## APPENDIX 5:   RATES OF SEXUALLY TRANSMITTED DISEASES IN THE UK AND US, 1995–2004

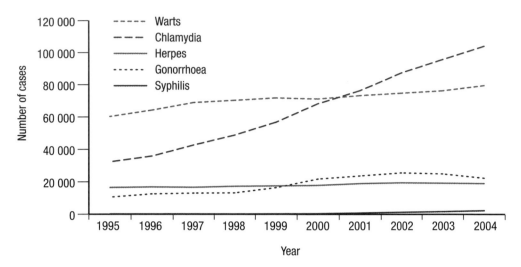

**APPENDIX 5.1**  Rates of sexually transmitted diseases in the UK 1995–2004.

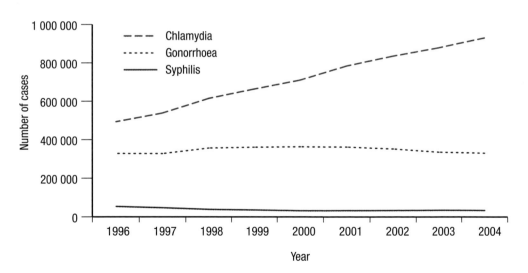

**APPENDIX 5.2**  Rates of sexually transmitted diseases in the United States 1995–2004.

# Index